HEALING
IN HYPNOSIS

HEALING
IN HYPNOSIS

THE SEMINARS, WORKSHOPS, AND LECTURES OF MILTON H. ERICKSON

VOLUME I

By
Milton H. Erickson

Edited by
Ernest L. Rossi
Margaret O. Ryan
Florence A. Sharp

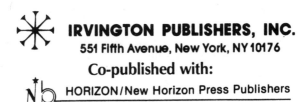

IRVINGTON PUBLISHERS, INC.
551 Fifth Avenue, New York, NY 10176
Co-published with:
HORIZON/New Horizon Press Publishers

Library of Congress Cataloging in Publication Data

Erickson, Milton H.
    Healing in hypnosis.

    (The Seminars, workshops, and lectures of
Milton H. Erickson ; v. 1)
    Bibliography: p.
    Includes index.
    1. Hypnotism.   2. Hypnotism--Therapeutic use.
I. Rossi, Ernest Lawrence.   II. Sharp, Florence A.,
1913-   . III. Ryan, Margaret O'Loghlin.   IV. Title.
V. Series: Erickson, Milton H. [Selections. 1982]
RC495.E713   154.7   82-6632
ISBN 0-8290-0739-3

Printed in the United States of America

CONTENTS

Acknowledgments ... vii

Prefatory Notes ... ix

Preface ... xi

Introduction ... 1
Milton H. Erickson: A Biographical Sketch

Part I ... 61
Utilizing Unconscious Processes in Hypnosis ... 61
Demonstration: Trance in Therapy and
Everyday Life ... 76

Part II ... 99
Therapeutic Uses of Altered Orientation in Hypnosis

Part III ... 161
Experiential Learnings: The Basis for Hypnotic Behavior

Part IV ... 217
An Introduction to the Study and Application of
Hypnosis in Pain Control

Bibliography ... 279

Milton H. Erickson: A Photographic Portfolio ... 283

Index ... 303

ACKNOWLEDGMENTS

We wish to express our appreciation and gratitude to Elizabeth Erickson and the Erickson family for contributing the treasured photographs presented in this volume.

PREFATORY NOTES

Regarding References

Because of the informal nature of the material, the editors decided to use footnotes rather than the standard APA format for referencing. To simplify frequent references to previous Erickson/Rossi volumes, only abbreviated titles are used in the text. Full publication information can be found in the bibliography.

Regarding the Typesetting

To indicate Erickson's frequent shifts of attention during demonstrations from subjects to audience and back to subjects, all verbatim trance material spoken directly to subjects is in bold face type, while his shifts of focus back to the audience are indicated by additional spacing and regular (Roman) type. (It should be noted, however, that although addressing the audience, many of Erickson's remarks are being directed to the subjects as forms of indirect suggestions.) Finally, any added commentary is indented.

PREFACE

This first volume of Milton H. Erickson's seminars, work-shops, and lectures has its beginnings in the efforts of many scholars and professionals in psychiatry, dentistry, psychology, and education to collect and preserve his teachings in the area of hypnosis, human development, and hypnotherapy. Since Erickson lectured and taught his fellow professionals in seminars and workshops for almost fifty years in all parts of the globe and under all sorts of circumstances, the process of editing his spoken words into written form has been a formidable task—one that has overwhelmed many scholarly and group efforts to systematize and publish an authoritative version of his work.

Florence Sharp, Ph.D., who was one of Erickson's closest students, initiated this current project back in the 1960s when she began to collect from former students and professionals who had sponsored Erickson's lectures and workshops, whatever audio and written records they had of Erickson's teachings. With the cooperation of many members of The American Society of Clinical Hypnosis and its component societies, she collected dozens of audio tapes and began the process of transcribing them into rough drafts of typed material.

For a generation, Florence built her collection until many filing cabinets and fireproof safes throughout her home bulged with a greater and greater accumulation of materials which she heroically catalogued and bravely tried to keep organized. She made multiple copies of everything so that the Ericksons and a few others might work on them. Alas, the task of trying to encompass and digest this vast accumulation was too much for any individual or committee. A generation of scholars grew old and essentially gave up trying to systematize all the material for publication in a thoroughly scholarly fashion.

When the senior editor (Ernest Rossi) discussed the problem with Erickson in the 1970s, it was decided that Erickson's papers should be published first as a separate set of volumes *(The Collected Papers of Milton H. Erickson on Hypnosis)*. Although that set of four volumes contained many previously unpublished papers (and excerpts from a few tapes to amplify some of his previously published papers), they were all highly focused and written in the traditional manner of scholarly papers.

Erickson's lectures and demonstrations in seminars and workshops before his fellow professionals, however, were not of a neatly systematic and scholarly nature. They were usually spontaneous, wide-ranging presentations with only a very general theme to guide them. The special interests, needs, and questions from each group frequently generated fresh insights and ingenius, unpremeditated demonstrations of hypnosis and hypnotherapy. All contributed to a significant paradigmatic shift from the older authoritarian techniques of hypnosis to the more permissive approaches pioneered by Erickson.

Because of this very informal nature of Erickson's lectures and demonstrations, it was decided that they could be published most appropriately without the scholarly trappings that might only distort their spontaneous quality. Previous efforts to bring them to publication probably failed precisely because the editors presumed to do too much: It is not yet possible to systematize Erickson's creative contributions in any highly organized and theoretical manner. Erickson loved the free play of nature. Although he began his research career with highly organized and controlled laboratory investigations of the nature of hypnosis and hypnotic phenomena, he gradually came to prefer "field experiments" where he could utilize naturally occurring events to explore the nature of altered states and hypnotherapeutic approaches. He spoke and taught in this same naturalistic manner. His verbal teachings, then, could only be presented in an informal manner, as we are doing in these volumes.

Just how informal? Well, as Rossi and Ryan browsed through Florence Sharp's collection, they found that one presentation was clearer or better organized than another from the same time period. When the same general material was covered in both presentations, the clearer one was naturally chosen for publication. By this method of paired comparisons, they gradually selected the best four or five presentations for each five-year period in the 1950s through the 1970s. Each of these selections is becoming the basis for a volume in this series.

Margaret Ryan, who worked personally with Erickson and did editing work on all but one of the Erickson-Rossi volumes, then took the favored manuscripts in rough draft form and, in close collaboration with Rossi, edited the spoken word into written sentences, paragraphs, and appropriate sections with subject headings.* We tried to use Erickson's words as exactly as possible, but frequent minor changes were required to translate his extemporaneous delivery into a smoothly readable and editorially correct form. In any rephrasing, however, the primary concern was to retain Erickson's unique style of presentation. On occasion it was necessary to delete material when it was either repeated too often or was lost in the audio recording.

Once these lightly edited versions were prepared, Rossi finished the editing by studying each presentation as a whole unit, seeking the main themes so that he could create a general title for the entire presentation. Rossi then added footnotes here and there to tie the material to previously published Ericksonian material. Rossi and Ryan cooperated in occasionally adding necessary explanatory material to the text to help the reader through those inevitable disjunctions of understanding that crop up between the spoken and written word.

It was found convenient to publish first these four presenta-

*The Index has been carefully keyed to these subject headings, and is the best guide to reaching the specific contents of each volume in this series.

tions from the early 1960s. In each succeeding volume we will concentrate on a time period of perhaps five years. To attempt a more formal organization by time or subject frames of reference is more than we can handle. We will continue to rely on footnotes to tie the whole evolving project together as it takes place.

The publication of these spontaneous talks and lectures, then, is itself another spontaneous process with only the experience and good will of the editors and the advice of our fellow professionals to guide us. Copies of the original tapes and some rough drafts of the originally transcribed material will be placed with official organizations, such as The American Society of Clinical Hypnosis[1] and The Milton H. Erickson Foundation,[2] so that the scholars of the future can make a more detailed examination of our work.

Our aim is to present the material in an enjoyable and readable style. We are relying on Erickson's own penchant for repetition with creative variations to present his ideas and styles of thinking and experiencing in as valid a manner as is humanly possible at the present time.

Ernest Rossi
Margaret Ryan
Florence Sharp

[1] Address: 2400 East Devon, #218, Des Plaines, Illinois 60018.

[2] Address: 1935 East Aurelius Ave., Phoenix, Arizona 85050

INTRODUCTION

MILTON H. ERICKSON:
A BIOGRAPHICAL SKETCH
By Ernest Rossi

Early Family History

How can we draw a picture of the life of that wily American farm boy who had enough mischievousness to outfox tragic personal illness and become a genius in healing and hypnosis? Let us go back to the beginning as he himself loved to tell it—back to the saga of his pioneering parents, and the three-sided log cabin he was born in during the days of the covered-wagon West.

Milton liked to tell the story of how his father, Albert, left home in Chicago at the age of 16 with nothing more than a train ticket and the Viking spirit of his forefathers to gird him. He got as far west as his money could take him, and eventually found himself hitching a ride in the rolling green farmlands around Lowell, Wisconsin. Hearing that a local farmer needed help, Albert went straight to the farm and quickly saw what he liked: a shy, pretty girl peeping from behind a tree.

"Whose girl are you?" he asked. "I'm my daddy's girl," said she. "Well, you're my girl now," replied he.

And so it was. Albert worked for the farmer, and in 1891 when he was 21 he married the 19-year-old Clara.* Life was not

---

*Many years later their son, Milton, would find a satisfying identity from the small bit of Viking blood on his father's side and the small bit of American Indian blood on his mother's side. Milton felt his background gave him a deeply rooted connection to the "natural man," with his strength and endurance in the face of adversity.

1

easy for the young couple. Farming was always precarious in pioneering country and the young Albert found himself looking elsewhere for a living. Strangely enough, Albert's first job presaged what would become his unborn son's profession: He found himself with a year's contract to work as an attendant in a mental hospital, with only occasional time off to visit his wife at home.

Next the Viking spirit and the romance of prospecting in those feverish times drew Albert to the lure of the Nevada silver mines. The Erickson family now travelled across country by train and covered wagon to the tiny hamlet of Aurum, Nevada. The trip out West was a difficult one, fraught with the kinds of hardship typical of pioneering adventures: there were food and water shortages, bitter cold nights, and fierce wind storms to endure, not to mention the sheer physical stamina required to make the long trip.

Once arrived the family resided in a three-sided, dirt-floored log cabin (the fourth side was a mountain!) in a desolate area of the Nevada Sierras. Constantly hindered by a shortage of supplies, the pioneers became quite skillful at transforming what was available into what was needed. Albert and Clara loved to tell how whisky bottles were used for jelly jars—one could remove the jelly with a knife—so that the scarcer, wider-mouthed jars could be used for other canned goods. Certainly growing up in this kind of resourceful environment helped form the prototype for what would eventually characterize Milton's highly innovative approaches to therapy: that of creatively utilizing whatever was available within the person to bring about change and healing.

This period of the Erickson family history was recorded by Don Ashbaugh in a chapter entitled "Give Me Back My Yesterdays," from his book *Nevada's Turbulent Yesterday* (Los Angeles: Westernlore, 1963). A week before his ninetieth birthday, on March 25, 1959, Albert Erickson wrote down some of his memories of camp life which Ashbaugh incorporated into his chapter: [The speaker being quoted in the opening paragraphs is Albert.]

2

"Aurum was not a rowdy camp. It was a happy little community where the miners and ranchers had good relationships. It had the only post office and store in the area. We had service on three stages a week.

"The miners always were welcome at homes of ranchers, with Aurum folks always happy to host visitors from the valley when they came for mail and supplies. Consequently, what few social events that were held, brought a mingling of the residents."

The families lived in log houses with dirt floors. Mrs. Paul Raddatz and her brother, Dr. Milton H. Erickson, were both born in the Erickson cabin. She described it as follows: "The house and cabin consisted of two large rooms, plus smaller bedrooms. The back had the mountain for a wall. The floors were dirt and all water was dumped on the floor to keep dust from forming. It did not get muddy due to the mineral content in the dirt." (pp. 327-329)

When the Erickson children reached school age, the family decided to return to Wisconsin and bought the farm where the young Milton spent his formative years. Fifty years later his parents were able to return to visit their beloved Aurum home. Their daughter recorded the scene, and Ashbaugh quoted her narration in his book as follows:

"The white-haired man [Albert] sat tensely erect in the car. His blue eyes scanned the mountain range. After forty-five years he was going back to the ghost camp of Aurum where he had mined silver for thirteen years.

"Suddenly he pointed and said sharply, 'That's it, that one with the basalt outcropping.' His wife looked closely and said slowly, 'No, I don't think so.' But the old man clung stubbornly to his decision.

"Shifting the car into low gear, it crawled slowly over a sort of jeep trail and after four miles lurched up a hummock to park at a site where a few old logs remained as mute evidence of a building having once occupied the spot.

"With an alacrity that belied his 86 years, he leaped from the car and excitedly proclaimed, 'This is it, this is the remains of the old stamp mill. See, here is part of a crucible. This is Aurum, Clary.'

"But 'Clary' continued to be skeptical. 'It doesn't look right, it's too steep. Where was Anderson's house? No, but wait, show me the cemetery and I'll believe.'

"'To heck with the cemetery,' the old man said sharply, 'I know my mountain.' A bewildered look passed over his face, the look of excitement was dulled as he gazed about and said slowly, 'It's Aurum, but it's changed, our road up to the mines is overgrown, that sheepherder's wagon is sitting in what was Anderson's yard and only a little wall shows the site of the post office. It's my mountain—but the rest is truly a ghost camp."

"His mood changed again as he gazed across the valley and the eyes brightened as he remarked, 'The red hills, Clary, they are just the same, it's just the man-made things that are gone.'

"Then in a voice deep with emotion, he looked up toward the mountain peak and said, 'Oh God, as I look at these great rock formations, the lush valley, the great pines, I can only say—Give me back my yesterdays! And, if one wish could be granted, I'd like to spend my few remaining years out in a little cabin with this mountain standing guard and listen to winds blow down the canyons and whisper lullabies to make me sleep.'" (pp. 330–331)

The love of country and the pioneering spirit so evident in this early family history was still a characteristic aspect of Milton's personal identity when I knew him in the last decade of his life.

Erickson's Early Life: Constitutional Differences and Altered Perceptions

Since Erickson was born and raised in pioneering and rural farming country, there were few medical or educational facilities. "Schooling" was simple and basic, which may be why no one (apparently) noticed that the young Milton was experiencing the world in his own unique manner. Many of Erickson's earliest memories dealt with the ways his perceptions differed from others' due to several constitutional problems: for one, he was color-blind*; for another, he was tone deaf and could neither recognize nor execute the typical rhythms of music and song; and still another, he was dyslexic—a problem which was indeed perplexing to his childhood mind and which he only recognized and understood by hindsight many, many years later.

The misunderstandings, inconsistencies and confusions that arose because of these deviations from the common, everyday world view might have inhibited another person's mental functioning. In the young Milton, however, these differences apparently had the opposite effect: they stimulated wonderment and curiosity. More importantly, they led to a succession of unusual experiences which formed the foundation for a lifetime of research into the relativity of human perception and the problems that arose because of it; and into therapeutic approaches dealing with those problems.

One day, when he was in his early seventies, Erickson re-

---

*There is a common myth that Erickson could see only the color purple as a result of a rare type of color blindness. According to Betty Erickson, this was not true. Milton had a common type of red-green blindness called "dichromatopsia." Purple became his favorite color, but he probably perceived it as a kind of darkened blue. Betty suggests that he chose purple early on because at that time it was rarely used for garments—and Milton thoroughly enjoyed being different. Eventually purple became his own personal trademark.

counted and discussed some of those experiences with me as follows:*

As a six-year-old child Erickson was apparently handicapped with dyslexia. Try as she might, his teacher could not convince him that a "3" and an "m" were not the same. One day the teacher wrote a 3 and then an m by guiding his hand with her own. Still Erickson could not recognize the difference. Suddenly he experienced a spontaneous visual hallucination in which he saw the difference in a blinding flash of light.

Erickson: Can you imagine how bewildering it is? Then one day, it's so amazing, there was a sudden burst of atomic light. I saw the m and I saw the 3. The m was standing on its legs and the 3 was on its side with the legs sticking out. The blinding flash of light! It was so bright! It cast into oblivion every other thing. There was a blinding flash of light and in the center of that terrible outburst of light were the 3 and the m.

Rossi: You really saw a blinding flash of light? You saw it out there, you're not just using a metaphor?

E: Yes, and it obscured every other thing except a 3 and an m.

R: Were you aware you were in an altered state? Did you, as a child, wonder about that funny experience?

E: That's the way you learn things.

R: I guess that's what I'd call a creative moment

*Unless otherwise indicated, all following quotations are taken from "Autohypnotic Experiences of Milton H. Erickson," M.H. Erickson and E.L. Rossi, *Collected Papers,* Vol. I, pp. 108–132. Originally published by *The American Journal of Clinical Hypnosis,* July, 1977, *20,* pp. 36–54.

(Rossi, 1972, 1973). You experienced a genuine perceptual alteration: a flash of light with the 3 and the m in the center. Did they actually have legs?

E: I saw them as they were. [Erickson draws a simple picture of a cloud effect with a 3 and an m in the center.] And this excluded everything else!

R: Was this a visual hallucination? As a six-year-old child you actually experienced an important intellectual insight in the form of a visual hallucination?

E: Yes, I can't remember anything else pertaining to that day. The most blinding, dazzling flash of light occurred in my sophomore year of high school. I had the nickname in grade school and high school, "Dictionary," because I spent so much time reading the dictionary in the back of the room. Suddenly a blinding, dazzling flash of light occurred because I just learned how to use the dictionary. Up to that moment in looking up a word, I started at the first page and went through every column, page after page until I reached the word. In that blinding flash of light I realized that you use the alphabet as an ordered system for looking up a word. The students who brought their lunch to school always ate in the basement. I don't know how long I sat there completely dazzled by the blinding light, but when I did get down to the basement, most of the students had finished their lunches. When they asked me why I was so late in reaching the basement, I knew that I wouldn't tell them that I had just learned how to use the dictionary. I don't know why it took me so long. Did my unconscious purposely withhold that knowledge because of the immense amount of education I got from reading the dictionary? . . . .

E: I must have had a slight dyslexia. I thought I knew for an absolute fact that when I said "co-mick-al, vin-

7

gar, goverment, and mung" my pronunciation was identical with the sounds made when others said "comical, vinegar, government, and spoon." When I was a sophomore in high school, the debating coach spent a useless hour trying to teach me how to say "government." Upon sudden inspiration she used the name of a fellow student, "La Verne," and wrote on the blackboard, "govLaVernement." I read, "govlavernement." She then asked me to read it, omitting the La of La Verne. As I did so a blinding flash of light occurred that obliterated all surrounding objects including the blackboard. I credit Miss Walsh for my technique of introducing the unexpected and irrelevant into a fixed, rigid pattern to explode it. A patient walked in today trembling and sobbing, "I'm fired. It always happens to me. My boss always bullies me. They always call me names and I always cry. Today my boss yelled at me saying, 'Stupid! stupid! stupid! Get out! Get out!' So here I am." I said very earnestly and seriously to her, "Why don't you tell him that if he had only let you know, you would have gladly done the job much more stupidly!" She looked blank, bewildered, stunned, and then burst into laughter, and the rest of the interview proceeded well with sudden gales of laughter—usually self-directed.

R: Her laughter indicates you had helped her break out of her limited view of herself as a victim. A basic principle of your *utilization* approach is illustrated in your early experience with Miss Walsh. She utilized your ability to pronounce La Verne to help you break out of your stereotyped error in pronouncing *government*. (pp. 109–111)

Perhaps it was from the muddle of such perceptual difficulties that the young Milton learned to ask more searching questions than most children his age. An example: Before the age of 10, Milton wanted to know why his grandfather planted potatoes with the eyes up and always during a certain phase of the moon. He was not satisfied with the answer he received, and proceeded to design and execute his first controlled experiment: he planted some potato patches with the eyes in all directions and at different phases of the moon; the other potato patches he planted in accordance with his grandfather's method. Milton was very saddened when his grandfather would not believe that all the potato patches had produced the same results!

During this same time period Erickson's native cleverness was illustrated in the following incident that he recalled many years later. In it he recounts how he used a double bind to solve a problem, although, of course, the term had not yet been coined*:

> My first well remembered intentional use of the double bind occured in early boyhood. One winter day, with the weather below zero, my father led a calf out of the barn to the water trough. After the calf had satisfied its thirst, they turned back to the barn, but at the doorway the calf stubbornly braced its feet, and despite my father's desperate pulling on the halter, he could not budge the animal. I was outside playing in the snow and, observing the impasse, began laughing heartily. My father challenged me to pull the calf into the barn. Recognizing the situation as one of unreasoning stubborn resistance on the part of the calf, I decided to let the calf have full opportunity to resist since that was what it apparently wished to do. Accordingly I presented the calf with a double bind by seizing it by the tail and pulling it away from the barn, while my father continued to pull it inward. The calf promptly chose to resist the weaker of the two forces and dragged me into the barn. (p. 412)

*From "Varieties of Double Bind," M. H. Erickson and E. L. Rossi, *Collected Papers*, Vol. I, pp. 412-429. Originally published by *The American Journal of Clinical Hypnosis*, January, 1975, *17*, pp. 143-157.

Polio and the Self-Discovery of Hypnosis

If ever a person lived out the archetype of the wounded physician—one who learns to heal others by first healing oneself—that person was Milton H. Erickson. The most formative experience in Erickson's early life was his first bout with polio at the age of 17 (his second bout occurred at the age of 51). In the following conversation he recounts that life crisis and his experiences of the altered perceptual states that he later recognized as a type of authohypnosis:

> E: As I lay in bed that night, I overheard the three doctors tell my parents in the other room that their boy would be dead in the morning. I felt intense anger that anyone should tell a mother her boy would be dead by morning. My mother then came in with as serene a face as can be. I asked her to arrange the dresser, push it up against the side of the bed at an angle. She did not understand why, she thought I was delirious. My speech was difficult. But at that angle by virtue of the mirror on the dresser I could see through the doorway, through the west window of the other room. I was damned if I would die without seeing one more sunset. If I had any skill in drawing, I could still sketch that sunset.

> R: Your anger and wanting to see another sunset was a way you kept yourself alive through that critical day in spite of the doctors' predictions. But why do you call that an autohypnotic experience?

> E: I saw that vast sunset covering the whole sky. But I know there was also a tree there outside the window, but I blocked it out.

> R: You blocked it out? It was that selective perception that enables you to say you were in an altered state?

> E: Yes, I did not do it consciously. I saw all the sunset,

but I didn't see the fence and large boulder that were there. I blocked out everything except the sunset. After I saw the sunset, I lost consciousness for three days. When I finally awakened, I asked my father why they had taken out that fence, tree, and boulder. I did not realize I had blotted them out when I fixed my attention so intensely on the sunset. Then, as I recovered and became aware of my lack of abilities, I wondered how I was going to earn a living. I had already published a paper in a national agricultural journal: "Why Young Folks Leave the Farm." I no longer had the strength to be a farmer, but maybe I could make it as a doctor.

R: Would you say it was the intensity of your inner experience, your spirit and sense of defiance, that kept you alive to see that sunset?

E: Yes, I would. With patients who have a poor outlook you say, "Well, you should live long enough to do this next month." And they do. (pp. 111-112)

Just how Milton recovered is one of the most fascinating stories of self-help and discovery I have ever heard. When he awakened after those three days he found himself almost totally paralyzed: he could hear very acutely; he could see and move his eyes; he could speak with great difficulty; but he could not otherwise move. There were no rehabilitation facilities in the rural community, and for all anyone knew he was to remain without the use of his limbs for the rest of his life. But Milton's acute intelligence continued to probe. For example, he learned to play mental games by interpreting the sounds around him as he lay in bed, all day: by the sound of just how the barn door closed and how long it took the footsteps to reach the house, he could tell who it was and what mood he or she was in.

Then came that critical day when his family forgot that they had left him alone, tied into the rocking chair. (They had fashioned a kind of primitive potty for Milton by cutting a hole in the seat of the chair.) The rocking chair was somewhere in the middle of the room with Milton in it, looking longingly at the window, wishing he were closer to it so that he could at least have the pleasure of gazing out at the farm. As he sat there, apparently immobile, wishing and wondering, *he suddenly became aware that his chair began to rock slightly.* What a momentous discovery! Was it an accident? Or did his wishing to be closer to the window actually stimulate some minimal body movement that set the chair to rocking?!

This experience, which probably would have passed unnoticed by most of us, led the 17-year-old lad into a feverish period of self-exploration and discovery. Milton was discovering for himself the basic ideomotor principle of hypnosis discussed by Bernheim a generation earlier: *exercising the thought or the idea of movement could lead to the actual experience of automatic body movement.*

In the weeks and months that followed, Milton foraged through his sense memories to try to relearn how to move. He would stare for hours at his hand, for example, and try to recall how his fingers had felt when grasping a pitchfork. Bit by bit he found his fingers beginning to twitch and move in tiny, uncoordinated ways. He persisted until the movements became larger and until he could consciously control them. And how did his hand grasp a tree limb? How did his legs, feet, and toes move when he climbed a tree?

These were not merely exercises in imagination; they were exercises in the activation of real sense memories—memories that sufficiently restimulated his sensory-motor coordination to enable him to recover. This is made clear in the following conversation with him:

> E: One of my first efforts was to learn relaxation and building up my strength. I made chains out of rubber bands so I could pull against certain resistances. I went through that every night and all the exercises I could. Then I learned I could walk to induce fatigue to get rid of the pain. *Slowly I learned that if I could think about walking and fatigue and relaxation, I could get relief.*

> R: Thinking about walking and fatigue was just as

effective in producing pain relief as the actual physical process?

E: Yes, it became effective in reducing pain.

R: In your self-rehabilitative experiences between the ages of 17 and 19 you learned from your own experience that you could use your imagination to achieve the same effects as an actual physical effort.

E: An *intense memory* rather than an imagination. You remember how something tastes, you know how you get a certain tingle from peppermint. As a child I used to climb a tree in a wood lot and then jump from one tree to another like a monkey. I would recall the many different twists and turns I made in order to find out what are the movements you make when you have full muscles.

R: You activated real memories from childhood in order to learn just how much muscle control you had left and how to reacquire that control.

E: Yes, you use real memories. At 18 I recalled all my childhood movements to help myself relearn muscle coordination. (pp. 112-113)

But something more than introspection was required for his recovery: external observation. At that time, fortunately, his youngest sister, Edith Carol, was just learning to walk. Milton began a campaign of daily watches in which he observed her (primarily unconscious) patterns of learning to walk so that he might copy them consciously—and thereby retrain his own body to do the same. In an unpublished conversation, he says of this period:

I learned to stand up by watching baby sister learn to stand up: use two hands for a base, uncross your legs, use the knees for a wide base, and then put more pressure on one arm and hand to get up. Sway back and forth to get balance. Practice knee bends and keep balance. Move head after the body balances. Move hand and shoulder after the body balances. Put one foot in front of the other with balance. Fall. Try again.

After eleven months of this intensive self-training, Milton was still on crutches but rapidly learning an increasingly economical limp that would put the least strain on his body.

College and Medical Training Years

At this point Milton was still not aware that his self-recovery via relaxation, sense-memory, and acute observation would be the foundation for his future work as the world's most innovative hypnotherapist. His body was recovering but was still weak, and he could not walk without the aid of crutches. After his freshman year at the University of Wisconsin, he was advised by a physician to spend a summer in nature to heal and strengthen his body. Not one to choose easy goals for himself, Milton decided a canoe trip might be just the thing.

Without the financial resources to guarantee a comfortable trip, Milton prepared to embark on his journey with only $4.00 in hand and, hopefully, a friend at his side. Since his ability to handle a canoe was marginal at best (imagine struggling to get a canoe in and out of water while jostling a pair of crutches at the same time!), it seemed obvious that a companion would not only be desirable but necessary. At the last minute, however, his friend decided not to go, so the undaunted Milton set out on his scheduled departure day quite alone. (He sensibly spared Albert and Clara the information that he, their inexperienced and handicapped son, was going to be riding the rapids unaided.) Armed with two weeks' supply of food, the necessary cooking gear, a tent, and a number of textbooks, Milton set off downstream with the idea that he would proceed in that direction until it was time to begin the return trip. Setting a specific destination, he believed, would only make the journey a laborious one.

Milton had many anecdotal adventures along the way. In the

very beginning of his trip he set out early one morning to fish for supplies but could not get back out of the lake until late that afternoon: high winds together with his own physical limitations resulted in several hours of challenging struggle. Soon, however, Milton became quite clever at indirectly soliciting the aid of others in those situations he simply could not handle alone—portaging a dam here and there, and so on. He also managed to get himself invited to many a camper's meal, where he would spend the afternoon swapping adventure tales over a picnic table and a lot of food. It seemed that picnickers and campers always found something interesting and intriguing about young Milton. (Indeed, this arranging of situations so that people would "spontaneously" help him had earned Milton the nickname of "Eric the Badger" from his Wisconsin classmates. How often they had found themselves, half in mirth and half in rue, giving this curious but shrewd farm boy certain advantages in competitive situations without ever quite knowing why!)

At several points throughout his journey, Milton took on temporary jobs with local farmers, thereby earning enough money to replenish his provisions. He also discovered that his cooking ability was a negotiable asset: he managed to earn his board for a 250-mile segment of the trip simply by cooking for two young men on a summer adventure similar to his own.

By the time Milton began the return trip, his muscular capacity had increased to the point where he was able to make headway against the river current, and, more importantly, to portage the canoe unaided. By the end of the ten-week trip, his list of accomplishments was even more impressive: he had covered 1,200 river miles, relying solely on his own ingenuity and resourcefulness; he had begun the trip with $4.00 and ended it with $8.00; he had begun the trip on crutches and ended it with only a slight (but permanent) limp; and finally, he had begun the trip a frail lad in ailing health and he had ended it a robust young man with a new sense of confidence, pride, and personal independence.

Thus exhilarated and strengthened by the summer's heroic

idyll, Milton returned to college bursting with energy and determination to make up for the earlier gaps in his rustic education. How to do this? By taking on the journalistic world. Earlier he had worked at a sitting-down job at the local cannery to help finance his college education, but now he felt ready for better things:

E: I was forever observing. I'll tell you the most egotistical thing I ever did. I was 20 years old, a first-semester sophomore in college, when I applied for a job at the local newspaper, *The Daily Cardinal,* in Wisconsin. I wanted to write editorials. The editor, Porter Butz, humored me and told me I could drop them off in his mail box each morning on my way to school. I had a lot of reading and studying to do to make up for my barren background in literature on the farm. I wanted to get a lot of an education. I got an idea of how to proceed by recalling how, when I was younger, I would sometimes correct arithmetic problems in my dreams.

My plan was to study in the evening and then go to bed at 10:30 p.m., when I'd fall asleep immediately. But I'd set my alarm clock for 1:00 a.m. I planned that I would get up at 1:00 a.m. and type out the editorial and place the typewriter on top of the pages and then go back to sleep. When I awakened the next morning, I was very surprised to see some typewritten material under my typewriter. I had no memory of getting up and writing. At every opportunity I'd write editorials in that way.

I purposely did not try to read the editorials but I kept a carbon copy. I'd place the unread editorials in the editor's box and every day I would look in the paper to see if I could find one written by me, but I couldn't. At the end of the week I looked at my carbon copies. There were three editorials, and all three had been published. They were mostly about the college and its relation to the community. I had not recognized my own work when it was on the printed page. I needed the carbon copies to prove it to myself.

R: Why did you decide not to look at your writing in the morning?

E: I wondered if I could write editorials. If I did not recognize my words on the printed page, that would tell me there was a lot more in my head than I realized. Then I had my proof that I was brighter than I knew. When I wanted to know something, I wanted it undistorted by somebody else's imperfect knowledge. My roommate was curious about why I jumped up at 1:00 a.m. to type. He said I did not seem to hear him when he shook my shoulder. He wondered if I was walking and typing in my sleep. I said that must be the explanation. That was my total understanding at the time. It was not till my third year in college that I took Hull's seminar and began my research in hypnosis.

R: Would this be a practical naturalistic approach for others to learn somnambulistic activity and autohypnosis? One could set an alarm clock to awaken in the middle of sleep so one could carry out some activity that could be forgotten. Would this be a way of training oneself in dissociative activity and hypnotic amnesia?

E: Yes, and after a while they would not need the alarm clock. I have trained many students this way. (pp. 114–115)

Much as the young Milton seemed the master of his fate from such early experiments with his own unconscious, there were even greater lessons to be learned. The following is an example of how this young rural American began to form his identity as a physician:

E: I had a very bitter experience early in medical school. I was assigned to examine two patients. The first was a 73-year-old man. He was in every way an undesirable bum, alcoholic, petty thief, supported by the public

17

his entire life. I was interested in that kind of life, so I took a careful history and learned every detail. He obviously had a good chance of living into his 80's. Then I went to see my other patient. I think she was one of the most beautiful girls I had ever seen—charming personality and highly intelligent. It was a pleasure to do a physical on her. Then, as I looked into her eyes, I found myself saying I had forgotten a task, so I asked to be excused and I would return as soon as possible. I went to the doctor's lounge and I looked into the future. That girl had Bright's disease, and if she lived another three months she'd be lucky. Here I saw the unfairness of life. A 73-year-old bum that never did anything worthwhile, never gave anything, often destructive. And here was this charming, beautiful girl who had so much to offer. I told myself, "You'd better think that over and get a perspective on life because that's what you're going to face over and over again as a doctor: the total unfairness of life."

R: What was autohypnotic about that?

E: I was alone there. I know others came in and out of the lounge but I was not aware of them. I was looking into the future.

R: How do you mean? Were your eyes open?

E: My eyes were open. I was seeing the unborn infants, the children who were yet to grow up and become such and such men and women dying in their 20's, 30's, 40's. Some living into their 80's and 90's and their particular values as people. All kinds of people. Their occupations, their lives, all went before my eyes.

R: Was this like a pseudo-orientation in time future? You lived your future life in your imagination?

E: Yes, you can't practice medicine and be upset emotionally. I had to learn to reconcile myself to the unfairness of life in that contrast between that lovely girl and that 73-year-old bum.

R: When did you realize you were in an autohypnotic state?

E: I knew I was as absorbed as when I wrote the editorials. I just let my absorption occur but I did not try to examine it. I went into that absorption to orient myself to my medical future.

R: You said to yourself, "I need to orient myself to my medical future." Then your unconscious took over and you experienced this profound reverie. So when we go into autohypnosis, we give ourselves a problem and then let the unconscious take over. The thoughts came and went by themselves? Were they cognitive or imagery?

E: They were both. I would see this little baby that grew up to be a man. (pp. 115-116)

At the time of this critical incident, Milton did not label the experience as autohypnotic. He was beginning to recognize, however, that some of the phenomena in his inner experiences were discussed by others under the rubric of hypnosis. This led to his first formal course of study with Clark L. Hull. Erickson later described this initial training as follows*:

During the 1923-24 formal Seminar on Hypnosis at the University of Wisconsin under the supervision of Clark L. Hull, the author, then an undergraduate student, reported for the discussion by the postgraduate students of the psychology department upon his own many and varied experi-

*From "Initial Experiments Investigating the Nature of Hypnosis," *Collected Papers*, Vol. I, pp. 3-17. Originally published by *The American Journal of Clinical Hypnosis*, October, 1954, *1*, pp. 152-162.

mental investigative findings during the previous six months of intensive work and on his current studies. There was much debate, argument and discussion about the nature of hypnosis, the psychological state it constituted, the respective roles of the operator and the subject, the values and significances of the processes employed in induction, the nature of the subjects' responses in developing trances, the possibility of transcendence of normal capabilities, the nature of regression, the evocation of previously learned patterns of response whether remote or recent, the processes involved in individual hypnotic phenomenon and in the maintenance of the trance state, and above all the identification of the primary figure in the development of the trance state, be it the operator or the subject. The weekly seminars were scheduled for two hours each, but usually lasted much longer, and frequently extra meetings were conducted informally in evenings and on weekends and holidays, with most of the group in attendance.

No consensus concerning the problems could be reached, as opinions and individual interpretations varied widely, and this finally led the author to undertake a special investigative project in October 1923. This special study has remained unpublished, although it was recorded in full at the time, as were many other studies. One of the reasons for the decision not to publish at that time was the author's dubiousness concerning Hull's strong conviction that the operator, through what he said and did to the subject, was much more important than any inner behavioral processes of the subject. This was a view Hull carried over into his work at Yale, one instance of which was his endeavor to establish a "standardized technique" for induction. By this term he meant the use of the same words, the same length of time, the same tone of voice, etc., which finally eventuated in an attempt to elicit comparable trance states by playing "induction phonograph records" without regard for individual differences among subjects, and for their varying degrees of interest, different motivations, and variations in the capacity to learn. Hull seemed thus to disregard subjects as persons, putting them on a par with inanimate laboratory apparatus, despite his awareness of such differences among subjects that could be demonstrated by tachistoscopic experiments. Even so, Hull did demonstrate that rigid laboratory procedures could be applied in the study of some hypnotic phenomena. (pp. 3–4)

Erickson's inevitable conflict with Hull stemmed from the early introspective healing work he had done and was still doing on himself. While this seemed to clash with the extravertedly oriented approach of the developing science of experimental psychology as represented by Hull, it did not clash with the concepts of introspection as developed by E. B. Tichener, Wilhelm Wundt, and W. B. Pillsbury. Erickson utilized such concepts to organize his initial laboratory studies of the internal dynamics of hypnosis and suggestion. His meticulous study of the inner forces and motivations of each individual subject was to become the pioneering hallmark of his "naturalistic," "permissive," and "indirect" approach to hypnosis. The best record of this early experimental research conducted while still a student was published later in two papers: "Initial Experiments Investigating the Nature of Hypnosis," previously cited, and "Further Experimental Investigation of Hypnosis: Hypnotic and Nonhypnotic Realities."*

A most original and distinguishing characteristic of these early investigations was Erickson's careful observation of the subtle interplay between the mental mechanisms of the awake state and those of the trance state. Erickson demonstrated how altered states and trance phenomena were also a normal part of everyday life. This understanding formed the underlying principle for his later studies of psychopathology as well as for his development of the naturalistic and utilization approaches to hypnotherapy. Erickson thus transformed the old authoritarian

*Collected Papers, Vol. I, pp. 18-82. Originally published by *The American Journal of Clinical Hypnosis,* October, 1967, *10,* 87-135.

view of hypnosis into a permissive and facilitative approach. No longer were rote suggestions automatically imprinted into the "blank" mind of a person in trance; instead, Erickson recognized the hypnotic trance state as one of dynamic complexity and individuality wherein the person's own capacities could be utilized to facilitate the healing process.

At the age of 23, while still a medical student, Erickson was married for the first time. He had three children by this marriage which lasted for 10 years before ending in divorce. I know very little about his personal circumstances during this period of his life, but from the few stray references Erickson made, it was very evident that he felt that the social and cultural isolation he experienced in his early years had left him with a certain social naivete and poor judgment about human relating. The pain and confusion he experienced over this first unhappy marriage, however, led him to a deepening resolve to focus his attention on understanding women and human relationships. He felt that he had grown up with many significant gaps in his understanding, and he had to work conscientiously throughout his adult life to fill them in. By the time I met him in his seventies, he held it as a cardinal principle that all normal adults had such gaps which they also had to fill in by continuing to learn about themselves throughout their entire lifetime.

Up to the time of his first marriage, Erickson had of necessity focused primarily on his own problems of physical illness and mental well-being. He now realized he would have to expand his attention beyond himself to the intricacies of loving and coping as well. This hard-learned lesson thus became another of the avenues of personal pain that led to a new area of pioneering professional work: Erickson was one of the first psychiatrists in the 1940s and 1950s to work with couples and families in the therapeutic encounter.

The Early Research Years

Upon graduating from the University of Wisconsin in 1928 with M.A. and M.D. degrees, Erickson entered into a general internship at the Colorado General Hospital and also served a psychiatric internship at the Colorado Psychopathic Hospital. He then received an appointment as Assistant Physician at the State Hospital for Mental Diseases in Howard, Rhode Island (1929-1930). His thesis for his Master's Degree had dealt with the feeble-minded, and he now expanded this work to explore the relationship among such factors as intelligence, marriage, abandonment, and crime. His findings were published by various medical, social, and legal journals in a series of seven papers between 1929 and 1931.

It wasn't until his next series of positions at Worcester State Hospital in Massachusetts (1930-1934), where he began as a junior physician and ended as Chief Psychiatrist on the research service, that he published his first paper dealing with hypnosis: "Possible Detrimental Effects from Experimental Hypnosis."* In this paper he dealt with the first task he had had to accomplish in a hospital and professional atmosphere that was initially hostile to what many regarded as a dark and fearful art: he demonstrated experimentally that hypnosis was a safe procedure.

During this early period hypnosis was still regarded as a form of sleep. With the popularization of Pavlovian theory, the sleep concept had been elevated into one of "cortical inhibition." But Erickson would have none of it. His own life experience led him to understand hypnosis as an altered state wherein subjects experienced an intense but more narrowly focused attention. This view is made clear in the following dialogue I had with Erickson when he was in his seventies, in which he recalled those early years:

E: In doing experimental hypnotic work with a subject in the laboratory I would notice we were all alone. The only thing present was the subject, the physical apparatus I was using to graph his behavior, and myself.

R: You were so focused on your work that everything else disappeared?

*Originally published by *The Journal of Abnormal and Social Psychology*, 1932, *37*, 321-327. In *Collected Papers*, Vol. 1, pp. 493-497.

E: Yes, I discovered I was in a trance with my subject. The next thing I wanted to learn was, could I do equally good work with reality all around me, or did I have to go into trance. I found I could work equally well under both conditions.

R: Do you tend to go into autohypnosis now when you work with patients in trance?

E: At the present time if I have any doubt about my capacity to see the important things I go into a trance. When there is a crucial issue with a patient and I don't want to miss any of the clues, I go into trance.

R: How do you let yourself go into such trance?

E: It happens automatically because I start keeping close track of every movement, sign, or behavioral manifestation that could be important. And as I began speaking to you just now, my vision became tunnel-like and I saw only you and your chair. It happened automatically, that terrible intensity, as I was looking at you. The word "terrible" is wrong; it's pleasurable.

R: It's the same tunnel vision as sometimes happens when one does crystal gazing?

E: Yes. (pp. 116-117)

These states of highly focused attention were not dissociated from normal consciousness. That is, Erickson was able to recognize that he had been in an altered state when he was in it, and he could recognize and remember the change when he came out of it. This was in contrast to other states of somnambulistic activity wherein he was completely dissociated, did not know he was in an altered state when he was in it, and had no memory of its contents when it was over—as, for example, when he wrote his student editorials. In the state of highly focused attention, however, Erickson could interact well with others and yet still be dissociated, as the following example from a much later stage in his career illustrates:

> Erickson now recounts a most amazing instance of when he went into trance spontaneously during the first sessions of his therapeutic work with a well-known and rather domineering psychiatrist from another country who was an experienced hypnotherapist. Erickson explains that he felt overwhelmed by his task but approached his first session with the expectation that his unconscious would come to his aid. He recalls beginning the first session and starting to write some notes. The next thing he knew he was alone in his office; two hours had passed, and there was a set of therapy notes in a closed folder on his desk. He then recognized he must have been in an autohypnotic state. Erickson respected his unconscious enough to allow his notes to remain unread in the closed folder. Spontaneously, without quite knowing how it happened, he went into a trance in the same way for the next 13 sessions. It wasn't until the 14th session that the psychiatrist-patient suddenly recognized Erickson's state. He then shouted, "Erickson, you are in trance right now!" Erickson was thus startled into normal awake state. He remained normally awake for the rest of the sessions. Erickson's profound respect for the autonomy of the unconscious is indicated by the fact that he never did read the notes he wrote while in autohypnotic trance during those first 14 sessions. The junior author recently looked at those faded pages and found they were nothing more than the typical notes a therapist might write. (p. 117)

By the end of his tour of duty at Worcester, Massachusetts, in 1934, Erickson's first marriage had also ended. He was 33 and the father of three young children he had to care for—at that time a rather unusual position for an unusual psychiatrist. When he accepted his next appointment at Wayne County General Hospital in Eloise, Michigan, however, he began a new and deeply searching chapter in his personal and professional life. And within a year he met Elizabeth (Betty) Moore who became his wife, his fellow researcher, and mother to his three children (and eventually to five more).

Erickson's appointment at Eloise—first as Director of Psychiatric Research (1934-39) and later as Director of Psychiatric Research and Training (1939-1948)—provided the locus for his major experimental research studies on the nature and reality of hypnotic phenomena. These ranged in scope from the carefully controlled laboratory experiments on hypnotic deafness and color blindness (with the help of his wife) to the investigation of hypnotically induced complexes and neuroses significant for clinical work. Erickson's fantastic abilities in utilizing minimal cues and indirect forms of suggestion led to the publication of a series of clinical papers on the experimental demonstration of Freudian mental mechanisms and the presence of unconscious processes in the "psychopathology of everyday life," as well as in severe psychiatric syndromes.

Although much of his work during this period supported psychoanalytic theory, Erickson never regarded himself as a Freudian, or for that matter, as a follower of any particular school. Indeed, he often decried the existence of the various schools of psychology and psychiatry because he felt the proponents too often demonstrated a premature rigidification of thought and method. Erickson realized that such rigidification (or "learned limitations") only inhibited further free exploration, and he himself remained atheoretical throughout his career. His was a genius of perception and communication that delighted in the study and therapeutic use of nature's ways; however, he felt no need to build theoretical webs of maya around those ways.

His reputation as a skilled observer and communicator grew from this early research phase of his career. He became an Associated Editor for *Diseases of the Nervous System* (1940-1955), and was much sought after as a consultant by the United States government in its cultural studies work and in relation to the war effort. Margaret Mead first consulted him in 1940 to help her review and analyze her films of spontaneous trance in the

Bali dancers. Erickson and Mead soon became close colleagues, and later served together on government projects during World War II that investigated the Japanese character structure and the effects of Nazi propaganda. Because these activities are still treated as classified information by the government, however, the full story about them remains for future scholars to unravel.

During the war years, Erickson served as a psychiatrist on the local draft induction board. This led to another of his clandestine activities—but this story can be told. Erickson would frequently write up incidents that took place at the draft board in anecdotal form and send them to H. C. L. Jackson, a columnist for *The Detroit News.* Jackson would edit them lightly and then publish them in his column as communications from one "Eric the Badger." This expanded to the point where Erickson was sending in all sorts of poignant and humorous stories which described diverse aspects of the human condition. Most of these were later published in book form by Jackson, and some even made it to the "big time": they were reproduced in such publications as the *Reader's Digest* column, "Life in These United States."

Erickson's early rural background and all-American identity were always very much evident in his penchant for communicating with the "average man." Throughout this time period he was called upon as a consultant and expert by the media through which he made strenuous efforts to clarify the public's understanding of hypnosis in the popular press *(Life Magazine, This Week Newsmagazine),* on radio, and through grassroots contacts in addresses to the Boy Scouts, the C.I.O., and high school graduation classes.

The Maturing Professional

Erickson's next significant career move was to accept the position of Clinical Director at Arizona State Hospital in Phoenix, Arizona (1948–49). The move to the dry and hot climate of Arizona was motivated in part by his painful reactions to the cold weather of Michigan and in part by the multiple allergies that had plagued him there.

The hospital superintendent in Arizona was John A. Larson,

Ph.D., M.D., an unusually gifted researcher and scholar who did much of the original research on the polygraph. He had fine intellectual rapport with Erickson, and together they hoped to build a progressive program of research and treatment. The Erickson family lived on the hospital grounds for the first year, but at that point Larson was called away to other duties and Erickson entered into private practice with his office in his home on Cypress Street in what is now downtown Phoenix.

The move into private practice despite Erickson's primary interests in research came about, once again, out of medical necessity. Although the dry heat and clean air of Arizona were helpful in reducing the muscle cramps and allergies he had experienced in the colder climates, Erickson was still prone to periods of vertigo, disorientation, and severe debility. The medical source of these problems was attributed to "residuals of poliomyelitis, possibly polioencephalitis."* However well he might be feeling, there was the everpresent possibility of pain and disability. Having an office in his home would permit him to take rest breaks between patients wherein he could reassert his autohypnotic control over the pain; it would keep his professional expenses to a minimum while making available the constant support and care of his wife; and he could be near his dogs and his children with whom he was always intensely involved as teacher, mentor, trickster, punster, wise storyteller, and loving companion.

Adopting this less stressful lifestyle turned out to be perspicacious, indeed. For within a few years, at the age of 51, Erickson experienced the rare medical tragedy of a second attack of polio. At this point in his life pain became a constant companion. This was in part due to the gradual and inevitable deterioration of muscle tissue that takes place with polio, and in part due to the residual effects of the unusual twists and pressures he had learned to put into his spinal column years earlier in his effort to hold as normal a body position as possible. In the following conversation, Erickson described to me the re-

*From a summary of a neurological examination by John A. Eisenbeiss, M.D., on December 12, 1960, and confirmed by Erickson's two personal physicians, T. E. A. vonDedenroth, M.D., and Marion Moore. M.D.

newed efforts he made to regain his functioning and control the pain through autohypnosis. Recovering from "Round Two":

R: Later, when you were 51, you incurred polio again. How did you help yourself?

E: By that time I could relegate things to my unconscious because I knew I had gone through all that before. I would just go into trance saying, 'Unconscious, do your stuff.' Learning to write with my left hand the first time was very laborious. The second time I got polio my right hand was knocked out again, and I found I had to use my left, which I had not used since around 19.

R: The sense memory exercises at 17 through 19 really helped you recover the use of your right hand and your ability to walk. When you were again stricken with polio at the age of 51, you had this base of experience to draw upon and left it up to your unconscious in autohypnotic trance.

E: At the present time (age 73) I have tried repeatedly to write with my left hand. [Erickson demonstrates how he now writes by holding the pen with his right hand but guides that hand with his stronger left hand.] I'm currently holding on very carefully to everything I can do with my right hand because I'd better keep whatever use I have as long as possible.

R: I see, that's why I see you peeling potatoes in the kitchen. You certainly are an example of the archetype of the wounded physician who learns to help others through his work in healing himself. This has been the story of your life. (p. 124)

Pain in daily life:

E: Yesterday I went into the house at noon to go to bed. I had to get rid of that agonizing pain here [in his back]. On my way to bed I asked my wife to prepare some grapefruit for me. The next thing I knew was that I went out and ate the grapefruit and rejoined you here in the office to continue our work. It was only then that I realized I did not have that horrible pain.

R: What did you do? Did you use autohypnosis to get rid of the pain?

E: I lay down on the bed knowing I'd better start to use autohypnosis in some way. But I don't know how I used it to get rid of the pain.

R: I see, it is a specific trance for that pain only.

E: It's a segmentalized trance.

R: Tell me more about that segmentalized trance.

E: S, with whom we worked yesterday, said her arms were numb. Not the rest of her body, only her arms. How do you get your arms numb? You segmentalize.

R: And the segmentalizing goes along with your conception of your body and not the actual distribution of sensory nerve tracts.

E: That's right. Pain is only part of your total experience, so in some way you must separate it off from your total experience. The pain was pretty agonizing here when I was in the office, so I went to bed with the intention of losing the pain. Then I forgot about losing it. When I came out here again, I suddenly realized I did not have the pain anymore.

R: Between lying on the bed and later eating the grapefruit the pain was somehow lost. But you don't know how or exactly the moment when.

E: That's right. I don't know how or exactly when, but I *knew* it would be lost. In losing it you also lose awareness that you did have pain.

R: In using autohypnosis you can tell yourself what you want to achieve but—

E: Then you leave it to your unconscious.

R: You cannot continue to question, "How am I going to lose it?" or think you can lose it consciously. This is very important in the use of autohypnosis. You can tell yourself what you want to achieve, but just exactly how and when it is achieved you have to leave to the unconscious. You must be content not to know how it is achieved.

E: Yes, that's right, because you can't know how it's achieved without keeping it with you.

R: As long as you are obsessively thinking about the pain, it is going to be there. You have to dissociate your conscious mind from the pain associations.

E: You must also have had an analogous experience such as this. (pp. 120–121)

Personally applied pain techniques:

E: At least for me physiological sleep will cause ordinary hypnosis to disappear. That means you should put your patients in a trance with instructions to remain in a trance until morning. In physiological sleep I simply let loose of the hypnotic frame of reference. I may awaken with pain, and I've got to reorient my frame of reference to a state of relaxation, a state of comfort, a state of well-being into which I am able to drift off into comfortable sleep. It may last for the rest of the night. Sometimes it

31

may last no longer than two hours, so I'm awakened and must reorient to comfort. Recently the only way I could get control over the pain was by sitting in bed, pulling a chair close, and pressing my larynx against the back of the chair. That was very uncomfortable. But it was discomfort I was deliberately creating.

R: It displaced the involuntary pain?

E: Yes, I drifted into sleep restfully; then I would awaken with a sore larynx.

R: My goodness! Why did you choose this unusual way of causing yourself pain?

E: Voluntary pain is something that is under your control. And when you can control pain, it's much less painful than involuntary pain. You know you can get rid of it.

R: It gets rid of the future component of pain (Erickson, 1967). You get rid of a lot of pain by displacement and distraction.

E: Right! Distraction, displacement, and reinterpretation.

R: Reinterpretation; can you give me an example of how you've used that?

E: Okay. I had very severe shoulder pain, and my thought was I didn't like the arthritic pain. You might call it a sharp, cutting, lancinating, burning pain. So, I thought of how a red hot wire would feel just as sharp and burning. Then it suddenly felt as if I really did have a hot wire there! The arthritic pain had been deep in the shoulder, but now I had a hot wire lying across the *top* of the shoulder.

R: So you displaced the pain slightly and reinterpreted it.

E: Yes, I displaced my attention so I was still having pain, but I didn't feel it all through the shoulder joint.

R: That was a voluntary reinterpretation, so it was more tolerable.

E: It is more tolerable, and then I got bored with it and finally forgot it. You can study that sensation only so long. When you've exhausted all that you can think about it, you finally lose the pain sensations. It wasn't until about four hours later that I recalled that I had had the hot wire sensation there. I couldn't recall just when I lost it.

R: So you make good use of forgetting too.

E: One can always forget pain. One of the things I don't understand about patients is why they continue to keep their tension and pain. (pp. 122-123)

Using memories to forget pain:

E: I get myself into a very awkward position on the bed so I cannot twitch too much. The twitching in my arms and legs and head jarred and aggravated me because I was having stabbing, lancinating, cutting pains. First here and there, very short, overall body discomfort. I was lying on my stomach with my feet elevated and my legs crossed. My right arm was under my chest, immobilizing me. I was recovering the feeling of lying prone with my arms in front of me, head up and looking at that beautiful meadow as a child. I even felt my arm short as a child's. I went to sleep essentially reliving those childhood days when I was lying on my stomach on the hill overlooking the meadow or the green fields. They looked so beautiful and so blissful and so peaceful. Or I see woods and forest or a slowly running stream of water.

R: You tap into those internal images from childhood when your body was in fact sound and comfortable. You thereby utilize the ideomotor and ideosensory process associated with those early memories to enhance your current comfort.

E: And when I was just learning to enjoy the beauty of nature. But an inactive beauty. It was the gentle movement of the grass in the breeze, but the grass itself was not putting forth the effort.

R: That image of a lack of self-directed activity led to a corresponding peacefulness within you.

E: Yes, and that filled my mind entirely. Then when I later came out here to see a patient, I let my intensity of observation take over completely in working with her.

R: You continued to distract yourself so the pain did not have a chance to recapture your consciousness. When you fill your mind with those early childhood memories, what is actually happening? Do you feel you are reactivating those associative processes in your mind and therefore, that simply displaces your current body pain?

E: Yes, and from a period of my life that is not very well informed, a simple and unsophisticated period. It allows a complete regression. I would have thoughts of my father and mother as they were *then!* Then I could have my own early feelings of being on the hill on the north side of the barn, etc.

R: And these feelings replaced the painful sensations you were having today?

E: Yes, I'm a visual type, so I use visual memories. [Erickson goes on to explain how he first explores a patient's early memories to determine whether they are predominantly visual or auditory. He then utilizes these predispositions in later trance work. One patient, for example, was able to distract himself from pain by focusing on the memories of the sound of crickets which he enjoyed in his childhood.] (pp. 123–124)

Another poignant dimension of his struggle (described by his wife, Betty):

> The unconscious may know more than the conscious mind, and should be left to develop its own learnings without interference, but it's not always plain sailing, and it may go about things in the wrong way.
>
> Some of [Milton's] experiences with pain control have been trial-and-error, with a good deal of *error*. For example, there have been many long weary hours spent when he would analyze the sensations verbally, muscle by muscle, over and over, insisting on someone (usually me) not only listening but giving full, absorbed attention, no matter how late the hour or how urgent other duties might be. He has absolutely no memory of these sessions, and I still don't understand them. I feel they were blind alleys, but perhaps they may have involved some unconscious learnings. Then again, maybe not. The reason I mention this is that I think many people might get discouraged when the unconscious gets lost temporarily in a blind alley. The message is "Hang in there. Eventually it will work through." (pp. 121–122)

Such intricate and idiosyncratic efforts to use autohypnosis for the relief of pain by one who was such an acknowledged master of hypnosis should dispel any notion of magic or mysticism regarding its nature and use. Throughout his life Erickson had little patience with the claims of parapsychology, with religious beliefs in miracles, or with popular fads about "psychic energy." Hypnosis for Erickson was a natural phenomenon that utilized ordinary psychological processes such as sense memory, forgetting, dissociation, and cognitive reinterpretation of belief systems. It usually required a great deal of training, intelligence, and work on the part of the therapist to help a patient achieve those seemingly miraculous results. But it only seems miraculous to the patient and casual observer because they do not know all the careful circumstances that are needed for the planned achievement of hypnotic effects. It is true that sociocultural circumstances will occasionally spontaneously fall into such arrangements where miracles appear to occur effortlessly and through some supernatural agency (i.e., at religious shrines or evangelical meetings, in the presence of colorful charlatans, etc.), but the ordinary therapist had better know everything possible about the sciences of psychology, human development, language, communication, and culture. Each patient is a unique microcosm who must be fully understood if an appropriate approach utilizing his or her individual potentials is to be synthesized. Although there are certain general principles of treatment to be followed, every hypnotherapeutic effort is, of necessity, experimental. With dedication, wit, and much practice, these hypnotherapeutic approaches can become almost "second nature" to the therapist, so that fine results are eventually achieved in a *seemingly* effortless manner.

The Leadership Years

Working in his home did not mean that Erickson was retiring to the sidelines. On the contrary, as soon as he recovered from the second bout of polio he found himself with enough extraverted energy to begin the most colorful and rewarding period of his career as friend, therapist, teacher, consultant—and eventually as a national and world leader in clinical hypnosis.

Erickson now began to teach as a guest lecturer at various local colleges and at workshops for fellow professionals. In the early 1950s he took part in teaching psychologists, psychiatrists, and dentists at the hypnosis seminars in Los Angeles with Leslie LeCron and others.

During this same period he met Aldous Huxley, and the two men became fine intellectual companions. Huxley's unusually gifted mind experienced fascinating hypnotic effects under Erickson's guidance. They had planned to do a joint work on consciousness and altered states, but unfortunately their unfinished manuscripts were destroyed by a fire that completely consumed Huxley's California home. Erickson used notes from some of their hypnotic sessions, however, to later write one of his most ingenious and colorful papers: "A Special Inquiry with Aldous Huxley into the Nature and Character of Various States of Consciousness."*

In 1950 Dr. Linn Cooper became interested in the phenomenon of time distortion and recognized that hypnosis might be a useful tool for investigating the ways in which time perception could be manipulated. He contacted Erickson, who was very much interested in his ideas. Cooper went to Phoenix where he spent the next several months designing and executing experimental investigations of the use of hypnosis in time distortion, employing psychology students from Arizona State University as subjects. Cooper recorded on paper his experimental findings, to which Erickson added the clinical and therapeutic applications; *Time Distortion in Hypnosis* was published in 1954 (Baltimore: Williams and Wilkins), with Cooper and Erickson as co-authors.

The first edition eventually sold out and a second printing was considered. By this time, however, Erickson and his wife had done exciting experimental work on "time expansion" as contrasted with "time condensation," and a second edition that would include this new discovery seemed more appropriate. This was published in 1959 (same title and publisher), again with Cooper and Erickson as co-authors.

Erickson's work with Cooper began an important pattern of collaboration that now provided a much needed vehicle for the articulation and publication of his ideas and techniques. Although Erickson had done most of his early research alone, and

*Originally published by *The American Journal of Clinical Hypnosis*, July, 1965, *8*, pp. 14-33. In *Collected Papers*, Vol. I, pp. 83-107.

had certainly published many scholarly papers by himself, his' performance skills as a hypnotherapist and teacher seemed to absorb most of his energy in his mature and later years. This meant that the books were usually written by the collaborators, who were all desperately trying to understand *"How Erickson did it!"*

Until Erickson came on the scene, the whole field of clinical hypnosis had been in abeyance. There just weren't that many professionals using it: It seemed that the older, authoritarian techniques of hypnosis simply did not appeal to a democratic culture fitfully trying to find itself. In America, the only professional organization of any significance was The Society of Experimental and Clinical Hypnosis that was composed primarily of academicians who focused on research rather than practice. Into this vacuum came Erickson who, with his indirect permissive approaches utilizing insight and mental mechanisms, initiated an exciting renaissance in the clinical worlds of doctors in the fields of medicine, dentistry, and psychology.

The interest and demand for professional training now grew to the point where Erickson and a number of colleagues (Edward Aston, D.D.S., Seymour Hershman, M.D., William Kroger, M.D., Irving Secter, D.D.S., and others) founded The American Society of Clinical Hypnosis, with Erickson as its first President (1957–59). In addition, Erickson initiated *The American Journal of Clinical Hypnosis* and served as its Editor for the first decade (1958–1968). The Associate Editors of the journal included Bernard Gorton, M.D., Theodore Mandy, M.D., Margaret Mead, Ph.D., Aaron Moss, D.D.S., Frank Pattie, Ph.D., Irving Secter, D.D.S., and Andre Weitzenhoffer, Ph.D. The first volume of the journal included corresponding editors in Chile, Japan, and Uruguay. Its scope, clearly, was to be professional, clinical, and international.

Erickson was now embarked upon the busiest time of his life. He had a burgeoning family of eight children, an ever-growing progression of assorted dogs, and an expanding professional reputation as editor, consultant, and teacher. His range was extremely diverse: he was a consultant to such varied groups as the U.S. Rifle Team, to government agencies involved in studying aircraft accidents, and to outstanding athletes who sought to maximize their performance potentials through the use of hypnosis. His lecturing to professional groups expanded across the country, so that he was usually absent from home at least one week every month. He was toasted internationally when he gave hypnotic demonstrations in front of professional groups in many countries where, since he could not speak the languages, he invented the spectacular pantomime techniques of hypnotic induction. Erickson described how he developed these techniques in "Pantomime Techniques in Hypnosis and the Implications"* that begins as follows:

> In the early experiments done by this author on hypnotic deafness, verbal communication having been lost as a result of the induced deafness, the value of pantomime was recognized, used, and then replaced by written communications as easier.
>
> The Pantomime Technique as a hypnotic technique complete in itself resulted from an invitation to address an affiliated society of American Society of Clinical Hypnosis, the Grupo de Estudio sobre Hipnosis Clinica y Experimental, in Mexico City in January, 1959.
>
> Just before the meeting the author was informed that he was to demonstrate hypnosis as the introduction to his lecture by employing as a subject a nurse they had selected who knew nothing about hypnosis nor about the author and who could neither speak nor understand English— they already knew that I could not speak nor understand Spanish. They had explained privately to her that I was a North American doctor who would need her silent assistance and they informed her of our mutual language handicaps and assured her that she would be fully respected by me. Hence she was totally unaware of what was expected of her.
>
> This unexpected proposal to the author led to rapid

*From *Collected Papers,* Vol. I, pp. 331-339. Originally published by *The American Journal of Clinical Hypnosis,* July, 1964, 7, 64-70.

thinking about his past partial uses of pantomime by gesture, facial expressions, etc. This lead to the conclusion that this unexpected development offered a unique opportunity. A completely pantomime technique would have to be used, and the subject's own state of mental uncertainty and eagerness to comprehend would effect the same sort of readiness to accept any comprehensible communication by pantomime as is effected by clear-cut definite communications in the Confusion Technique. (p. 331)

Confusion, indeed! At times everyone seemed confused around Erickson: wife, children, friends, strangers, dogs, colleagues, patients, and officials of all sorts. Nature had visited vertigo, sensory disorientation, and confusion upon him, almost as a way of life, and from such intimate knowledge of it he now claimed confusion as a major tool of his method. He would use his unusual perspectives and intellectual brilliance to confuse his subjects and patients in order to (in my later formulation) depotentiate the limitations and rigidities of their conscious mental sets so that their creative unconscious might have a better chance of becoming manifest. He frankly admitted that he was being "manipulative in the same sense as when you put salt on food to manipulate your sense of taste." He believed, however, that the unconscious mind has ways of protecting patients and subjects in hypnosis: it would accept and utilize any manipulation the therapist offered that was in the best interests of the person, but it would invariably reject any that placed the person in jeopardy or that gave an unscrupulous operator an unfair advantage. Erickson believed strongly in such self-protective defense mechanisms of the unconscious during hypnosis, and although challenged on it many times by colleagues and researchers, maintained and reiterated this viewpoint consistently throughout his career.

The research process of clarifying Erickson's procedures began in 1965 when Jay Haley and John Weakland attended a weekly demonstration given by Erickson in Phoenix, tape-recording it as part of their research for The Communications Research Project (directed by Gregory Bateson). These men were a part of the famous group at the Veterans Hospital in Palo Alto, California, that introduced the concept of the double bind in their 1956 paper, "Toward a Theory of Schizophrenia."[1] In a discussion of Erickson's demonstration, which was published in 1959 as "A Transcript of a Trance Induction with Commentary," Haley and Weakland made the exciting discovery that Erickson was using double binds. In the following example, the subject, Sue, had experienced an initial light trance and was now awakening from a second trance:[2]

E: After you are awakened again, Sue—and I ask you about going into a trance, I want you to tell me that you weren't asleep the second time, that you were the first time. And you're most insistent on that, and you will repeat that, Sue, will you not?

W: Now by changing your "no" to the second one, you begin to get your acceptance catching up as you go along?

E: Yes. First I had her deny the first trance. Now I'm nullifying that denial.

W: By giving her another "no" to work on in the meantime.

E: And in order to work on the second negation, she's got to affirm the first.

[1] G. Bateson, D. Jackson, J. Haley, and J. Weakland, *Behavioral Science,* 1965, *1,* pp. 251-264.

[2] From "A Transcript of a Trance Induction," M. H. Erickson, J. Haley, and J. Weakland, *Collected Papers,* Vol. I, pp. 206-257. Originally published by *The American Journal of Clinical Hypnosis,* October, 1959, *2,* pp. 49-84.

H: A use of double binds! . . . .

E: Every manipulator works it on that basis, too. . . .
In order to deny one of them, she has to affirm the
other. The affirmation of one of them is the means of
denying the other.

H: That's a classic double bind you've got there. (pp.
218–219)

The pulling of that calf's tail had come a long way, indeed!

Erickson's extraordinary performance skills as a hypnotic
operator now led to an invitation to give a demonstration in
Ernest Hilgard's laboratory at Stanford University in 1958. The
demonstration was filmed in 16mm.* Seemingly with great
casualness, Erickson used confusion, minimal cues, and ideomotor movements to establish a "reverse set" that led the subject to acknowledge she was experiencing trance even though
her conscious mind did not recognize it. This demonstration is
one of the best visual records we have of Erickson's skill at the
height of his career in activating and utilizing mental mechanisms—a process which he himself believed constituted the
essence of the hypnotherapist's art. It was a quest for this skill
that now led a constant stream of professionals and researchers
to the door of Erickson's humble home office during the final
two decades of his life.

The Sage of Phoenix

That humble home office on Cypress Street was a human-
izing experience for all who crossed its threshold. Patients constantly tripped over agreeable dogs and children in the family
living room that also doubled as a waiting room. A basset hound
named "Roger" was so relaxed lying in the middle of the floor
that patients often fell into reverie and trance just by watching

---

*This film was later transferred to videotape and was used as a center-
piece for the third Erickson-Rossi volume *(Experiencing Hypnosis).*

him. Thus Erickson felt his work was made easier. Indeed, it wasn't so much a matter of doctor-patient relationships as of family-patient relationships. Children would draw pictures for patients, and little, sweet-nothing gifts of sentiment would be exchanged. The family always knew when a patient was feeling better or worse, and sometimes extreme treatment methods would even be carried out in their own backyard: on at least one occasion Erickson locked up the boots of an alcoholic patient so that he would not run away from the backyard where he was drying out—while cleaning up after the dogs and gardening to earn his keep! Another patient who had to be hospitalized was "adopted" by the family: after he was released from the hospital they gave him a dog that was kept at the Erickson home (since he could not keep it in his apartment), and he visited that dog and the family daily for years—even to this day continuing regular visits.

Since all elements of home, family, and therapy were so marvelously intermixed, it was only natural that Erickson began to use homilies and stories about the family—and particularly about the children's developmental stages of learning—as indirect suggestions to stimulate patients' own healing and growth processes. It was plain to all that this was The Family Man with the steadfast, homespun values of Middle America. And the humble fees he charged were yet another reflection of his use of the virtues of the Middle Way.

Visiting professionals were always slightly dazed as they tripped through this menage. Was this really the home of the world-famous Milton H. Erickson? Books, journals, and manuscripts were crammed into homemade bookshelves and overflowing from small, rustic tables onto American Indian-made rugs. And although the family had moved to a new home on Hayward Avenue in North Phoenix in 1970 where the office was in a slightly detached guest house, the situation was not really altered: Milton delighted in taking his colleagues into the main house to admire his continuously growing collection of ironwood carvings. The new quarters were equally cluttered with a prized array of treasures and pets.

Erickson's miniscule office (it measured 10-1/2 feet by

9-3/4 feet) was dominated by one of those solid wooden desks of dubious vintage pushed into one corner, with some metal filing cabinets and a few ill-matched, uncomfortable chairs placed here and there. Homemade bookshelves covered two walls and held books on hypnosis from many ages in many languages. The cement block walls were painted a pastel green, and there were purple artifacts of various hues all over (a purple phone, a hand-knitted doll caricaturing Erickson in his purple robe, assorted rugs, mobiles, and knicknacks of every design and clutter). A large poster cartoon of a "Dumb Bunny" with a cigarette dangling from his lips was pasted on the side of one filing cabinet; on top of another was a large stuffed badger staring quizzically at patients; and behind him was a picture of Clara and Albert Erickson looking down at one, clear and serene in their American gothic poise. On top of one bookcase were dozens (perhaps even a hundred) of small, ironwood carvings made by the Seri, a Mexican-Indian tribe that Erickson practically supported by purchasing so much of their output. On the walls hung degrees and honorary certificates in recognition of Erickson's contributions to many foreign societies of medicine and hypnosis. Half hidden on the side of one bookcase was a faked portrait of Sigmund Freud in a general's uniform. It was always a great jest for Erickson when a visiting professional, upon entering the office, stared at that portrait for a full minute or two before poor old abused Sigmund was recognized in his unusual context. Like most of Erickson's jokes, it was an indirect lesson with an important implication to the visitor's unconscious: you need to give up your usual modes of perception to recognize the new in this place.

Two colleagues—Seymour Hershman, M.D., and Irving Secter, D.D.S., who had been founding members of The American Society of Clinical Hypnosis—now collaborated with Erickson in writing a text for use at the teaching workshops conducted by the Society.* By this time Erickson had published over 100

*M. H. Erickson, S. Hershman, and I. Secter, *The Practical Application of Medical and Dental Hypnosis*. New York: Julian Press, 1961.

44

papers in scholarly journals that were not readily available, so a brilliant young psychiatrist, Dr. Bernard Gorton, took on the task of assembling a complete collection. He discussed the project in 1958 with Erickson, Jay Haley, and Andre Weitzenhoffer, but died suddenly before it was completed. The scholarly Weitzenhoffer, who had already published two excellent, academically oriented texts on hypnosis, then attempted to produce a complete edition of Erickson's work, with the addition of recorded lectures and commentaries. His considerable enterprise in this direction did not come to fruition, however, so it was agreed that Jay Haley would simply edit a single volume of the most important papers then available. This was published in 1967 as *Advanced Techniques of Hypnosis and Therapy: Selected Papers of Milton H. Erickson, M.D.* (New York: Grune and Stratton). Haley followed up this work with a deeply moving volume on Erickson's therapy with individuals, couples, and families called *Uncommon Therapy: The Psychiatric Techniques of Milton H. Erickson* (New York: Norton, 1973).

Meanwhile I—with my dogmatic slumbers undisturbed—had written my first book, *Dreams and the Growth of Personality* (New York: Pergamon, 1972) without any awareness of Erickson's existence. In that book I had introduced a new phenomenological approach to dreams as a source of consciousness and identity, and had proposed methods for continuing and better completing dreams during the therapy hour. I was blissfully ignorant of hypnosis, and in fact found myself mildly irritated when some patients, after experiencing their own dream reveries in therapy, wondered aloud if they had been in a hypnotic state. I maintained that they had not, and moreover, how could such a silly notion enter their heads! Surely I was no hypnotist!

Finally one elderly patient, a retired school teacher with erection problems, thrust the Haley volume of Erickson's selected papers into my hands with the clear implication that this, perhaps, was a better way. A better way! That volume seized me with such numinous intensity that I stayed awake for three days and nights unable to put it down. On the fourth day, still struggling to put it down by my bedside while yet trying to grasp the concepts in the paper on confusion techniques, I felt a dull thudding pain in my gut before finally falling into an uneasy sleep. Upon awakening the pain remained, and a physician diagnosed a condition of acute gastritis. Never before had I experienced a psychosomatic ailment. Now this! What to do?

In his next session with me, the school teacher happened to mention that he had learned from the telephone directory that Erickson was still alive and residing in Phoenix. What else to do?! After a preliminary letter, I proceeded straight to Phoenix to get cured of my incipient ulcer. I made the eight-hour car drive there and back for four sessions, always somewhat in a daze. At the end of the fourth session, Erickson gently observed that I was no longer experiencing symptoms, that I was not really coming as a patient any longer, and so he could no longer accept a fee from me.

I felt he was dismissing me forever, so I explained in a torrent of words that he had been doing *twenty years ago* what I hoped to be doing (via the methods of my first book) *twenty years from now*. A number of papers had been writing themselves in my mind each time I left a therapy session and drove back to Los Angeles. I then let loose with a fevered flue of points, perceptions, phrases, and paragraphs purporting to explain and integrate his work with this and that. He did not seem at all surprised and simply remarked that since he was my senior, he would be the senior author and I would be the junior author of any papers I actually published. Then I just wheeled him from the office back into the house and left.[1]

I met Erickson in March, 1972, and by the next year my first paper on his work, "Psychological Shocks and Creative Moments," was published in *The American Journal of Clinical Hypnosis* (1973, *16*, pp. 9–22).[2] From then on all our work

---

[1] Erickson was always in a wheelchair in that last decade of his life when I knew him—just like my grandfather and namesake, Ernesto Rossi, who had come to America as an Italian laborer and had dug the subways of New York, eating bananas and walnuts every day for lunch, before he had the stroke that crippled him for life.

[2] In *Collected Papers,* Vol. IV, pp. 447–464.

was collaborative, with he as the senior author and I as the junior. I began the regular practice of spending a week or so every month living in the Erickson guest house and tape recording his sessions with patients—as well as I could. (The heat of Phoenix required that an ancient air conditioner be on during most of the sessions; that, together with the din of traffic and dogs, left much to be desired in terms of audio recording quality. Because of this, none of these tapes could be used commercially.) I would record for a week, return home to transcribe the tapes by hand and have them typed up, and then on my next visit would discuss the transcriptions in detail with Erickson. I would then return to Los Angeles, have the original session and our discussion session typed side by side, and on the third visit read both to Erickson for any final corrections or comments.

The first book to come out of this pattern of working together was *Hypnotic Realities.* I was very uncertain of myself in this first volume, and was quite aware of the depth and breadth of Erickson's consciousness in relation to my own. I struggled for authenticity, wanting the book to reflect "pure Erickson" with as little interference from my own viewpoints as possible. Yet I had the nagging awareness that permissive as he was, Erickson still came from an older authoritarian world view wherein he was able to justify words like *manipulation* and *technique.* I, on the other hand, was squarely within the humanistic and transpersonal traditions of Carl Rogers, Abraham Maslow, and Roberto Assagioli. I loved concepts of *soul* and *higher consciousness,* had become a Jungian analyst years earlier, and loved studying all of humanity's mystical and religious strivings toward *cosmic consciousness.* * As a pure naturalist, Erickson, on the other hand, had no use whatsoever for religion, and he had only the typical professional's misunderstanding of Jung and thinkers like him. What was worse, Erickson was quickly learning to spoof me by periodically using my own terms (e.g., *psychosynthesis, growth, creative, the new)* with sly seriousness. He was starting to teach me by utilizing the concepts already in

*See *Cosmic Consciousness,* by M. A. Bucke. New York: Innes & Son, 1901. Republished by Dutton, 1967.

my own mind! I could only stop that by more or less shutting up on my own vocabulary and struggling to use his. But some translations and modifications were required. Although I could understand and appreciate his benign use of the words *technique* and *manipulate,* we agreed that the concepts of *indirect hypnotic approaches* and the *utilization* of mental mechanisms would be the more appropriate conceptualization. This is what led me to focus so intensely on illustrating, naming, and explicating the *indirect forms of suggestions* that could be used to *utilize* and *facilitate* the patient's own mental mechanisms and *growth processes* in a permissive manner.

Some of Erickson's colleagues formulated his early therapeutic approach in terms that were more reflective of his temperament and personality than is my formulation. Leonard Ravitz, M.D., who was one of Erickson's earliest medical students (and later did pioneering work in what he believes are the "electromagnetic-field correlates of Erickson's discoveries"[1, 2]), has provided the most succinct and pungently accurate assessment of Erickson's own early "off the record" attitudes and understandings about the reasons for the effectiveness of his work:[3]

> Among the many naturalistic-utilization techniques Erickson invented, often combined with ideomotor and ideosensory phenomena, were the "double-bind," the introduction of a systematic series of paradoxes to deepen the hypnotic state, the confusion technique,

[1] L. J. Ravitz, "Electrometric Correlates of the Hypnotic State." *Science,* 1950, *112,* p. 341.

[2] _____, "History, Measurement, and Applicability of Periodic Changes in the Electromagnetic Field in Health and Disease." *American Archives of New York Science,* 1962, *92,* pp. 1144-1201.

[3] From L. J. Ravitz, "Leaders in Contemporary Science." *Journal of the American Society of Psychosomatic Dentistry and Medicine,* 1981, *28,* pp. 3-7.

and *the short-term "benevolent ordeal."* The latter was reinforced by at least implicit suggestions that proper twists of *the paradoxically kind therapist's stick would bring about necessary behavior alterations;* while simultaneously, patients were permitted or even encouraged to continue their systematic behavior, the persistence of which placed them at a *disadvantage in controlling the therapeutic relationship.* Mitigation of symptomatic behavior brought about a dissolution of the "ordeal" component. Erickson deemphasized "insight" as an important, or even necessary, element in treatment. (p. 6) [italics added]

As if to correct my own tender-minded image of him, Erickson would occasionally remind me that there was a "steel fist in my velvet glove." Yet when Erickson's approach did miscarry, it was probably because his "therapist's stick," the "short-term benevolent ordeal," and the "disadvantage in controlling the therapeutic relationship" were more than some patients could tolerate. I was able to witness at first hand one such unfortunate encounter with a patient I had brought to Erickson for consultation. (It is only fair to say, however, that Erickson was already in his mid-seventies, weak and ill, when the following incident occurred.)

I had been unable to make any therapeutic progress with this patient. It seemed she rendered me ineffective by being too affable, friendly, and cooperative—yet there was no change in her symptomatology. I did not warn Erickson of this transference problem, and was amazed when he sensed her subtly seductive efforts from the moment she walked in the door. He would have none of it, and was rather brusque with her right from the start. She seemed affronted, but nevertheless brought him a "gift" of a turquoise necklace and presented it to him at the end of their second or third session. I was aghast at the serious struggle that then broke out: Erickson refused the gift by handing it back to her three or four times with polite, verbal protestations that it was too valuable for a therapist to accept; finally, with sharp determination she flung

49

it on the table in front of Erickson, who in turn weakly managed to fling it away once more with his palsied hand, so that it fell on her departing heels as she stalked out the door! Here I learned via direct experience the drawbacks and risks of using confrontation and authority as techniques: when they don't work, a complete severance of the therapeutic relationship can easily result.*

The indirectly authoritative aspects of Erickson's orientation were further manifested by his appreciation of Lawrence Kubie's characterization of his double bind *technique* as giving the patient only an "illusory choice." My humanistic orientation led me to nudge this concept of illusory choice closer to "facilitating real choice" as the essential therapeutic dynamic of Erickson's *approaches*. Thus I concluded *Hypnotic Realities* with a section entitled "The Facilitation of Human Potentials" that reads as follows:

> Throughout this volume we have touched upon the various means by which human potentials and unrealized abilities may be explored and facilitated during trance. Trance in this sense can be understood as a period of free exploration and learning unencumbered by some of the limitations of a person's previous history. It is for this purpose that Erickson developed so many unique approaches to hypnotic induction and trance training wherein a person's usual limitations could be altered momentarily so that inner potentials could become manifest. The great variety of these approaches can never become standardized because happy humans are never static and standardized. Everyone is an individual in a process of development. The hypnotic interaction reflects and facilitates this development in ways that are creative and surprising to fine observers who are able to recognize the fetters that bind human nature. They are ever eager to make available means of freeing and facilitating human development.

*See "Psychological Shocks and Creative Moments in Psychotherapy" (in Vol. IV of *Collected Papers)* for a further discussion of this issue.

They then wisely stand aside to watch and wonder about its ultimate course. (p. 313)

This standing aside to "watch and wonder" about the ultimate course of human nature is more characteristic of my own mentality and stands in contrast to how "Erickson deemphasized 'insight' as an important, or even necessary, element in treatment." Ravitz continues his assessment of Erickson as follows (op. cit.):

> Unlike many psychiatrists, especially the psychoanalysts, Erickson never succumbed to the temptation of shifting his inductive focus into theoretic gear, nor of blurring his many empiric contributions by breathing more deductive life into transitory, directly sensed data than they deserve. His writings demonstrate a punctiliously careful usage of terms, all of which maintain ordinary directly sensed meanings. He avoided the employment of fashionable, illogically formulated psychoanalytic constructs to *describe* directly inspected or introspected factors. His papers comprise beautifully written, lucid descriptions and observations—the development of the natural history stage of inquiry to its highest degree. (pp. 6-7)

Erickson was a lucid naturalist who felt no need to go much beyond the sense observations of what was immediately present. I required the philosophical idealism of the humanistic world view to guide me through the ethical shoals of the therapeutic encounter, and to motivate me with a sense of destiny. When Milton died, it was perhaps this unresolved contrast between our temperaments that brooded within me as an unconscious tension, and that has been resolved only now—almost two years after his passing—as I write these words to clarify and resynthesize once more my own separate identity.

Because of the shifts in conceptual emphasis, and because I did all the writing and made all the major decisions on the organization of our books, I felt I needed some outside, objective check before sending the first book, *Hypnotic Realities,* to press. This outside check was admirably provided by Andre Weitzenhoffer, who read the manuscript carefully and discussed its details with Erickson and myself for three or four days. As Weitzenhoffer later wrote in his Foreword to the book,

> Although theory is neither the strength nor focus of this book . . . Rossi has proceeded to unravel, sift, analyze, translate, organize, and finally integrate what must at first have seemed to him to be a bewildering collection of data. . . . Rossi has succeeded, I believe, in giving us an opportunity to see in a unique way what Erickson does through the latter's very own eyes. (pp. xviii–xix)

It was heartening to have as meticulous a mind as Weitzenhoffer's understand what I was trying to do: He gave me the strength to continue.

I was a lot more relaxed and confident writing the second Erickson-Rossi volume *(Hypnotherapy: An Exploratory Casebook),* and in the first four chapters I made an effort to outline the entire process of Ericksonian Hypnotherapy. In it I also introduced the concept of left and right hemispheric differences, which Erickson was immediately able to appreciate as a basic orientation for organizing and understanding his diverse approaches.

Our third book, *Experiencing Hypnosis: Therapeutic Approaches to Altered States,* was produced under the pressure of Erickson's rapidly failing health, and in fact was published posthumously. We originally planned to have chapters on Erickson's approaches to each of the major hypnotic phenomena (we only succeeded in the second and third chapters on catalepsy and ideomotor signaling), but under the circumstances we felt it was more important to publish the best of what we already had. We particularly wanted to publish the detailed explication of the 1958 movie in which Erickson had demonstrated the reverse set induction in Hilgard's laboratory, as well as the detailed examples of Erickson's permissive approaches to facilitating the experience of trance by the modern rational and skeptical mind.

Next Erickson had entrusted to me a large cardboard box

filled with unfinished manuscripts that I might edit for publication. These and our continuing taped sessions provided the basis for all of the papers we published in the 1970s. The contents of the box then inspired me to finally pull together a collection of all of Erickson's papers in the area of hypnosis—a total of four volumes, which we published as *The Collected Papers of Milton H. Erickson on Hypnosis*. The box also contained transcriptions of Erickson's taped lectures and demonstrations (collected by Florence Sharp) which he had given in seminars and workshops for professional groups during the 1950s and 1960s. I am currently assembling these for publication of, probably, three to five volumes (of which this volume is the first).

Of the thousands of professionals who visited, studied, and recorded Erickson in informal group demonstrations at his home office in Phoenix during the 1960s and 1970s,[1] I met and knew only a few. Many of these professionals are currently writing, editing, and publishing their own versions of his work. Milton would probably approve of most, the exceptions being those with any tendency toward sensationalistic views, and those with non-naturalistic (psychic or supernatural) concepts.

Most interesting at the current time are the ideas of Bandler, Grinder, and Delozier, who use their two-volume work (with a third projected) on *The Patterns of the Hypnotic Techniques of Milton H. Erickson, M.D.*[2] as one of the foundations for their new approach of *neuro-linguistic programming* (NLP). Much as I might be disconcerted by their use of the word *programming* in association with Erickson's essentially heuristic approaches, NLP does base itself, theoretically and practically, on two of Erickson's special contributions: his skills of linguistic and

---

[1] The videotapes of Herbert Lustig, M.S., are an example of Erickson's work at this time (available through Irvington Publishers).

[2] R. Bandler and J. Grinder, Volume 1. Palo Alto, Calif.: Behavior and Science Books, 1975; and J. Grinder, J. Delozier, and R. Bandler, Volume 2. Palo Alto, Calif.: Behavior and Science Books, 1977.

sensory-perceptual reorganization. Another researcher in the field, Paul Watzlawick, uses Erickson to elucidate the role of left and right hemispheric functioning,[1] while Jeffrey Zeig uses a concept of "reframing" in his edited version of a teaching seminar with Erickson.[2]

The common thread among all these contributors seems to be a new, parsimonious yet humanistic use of Occam's Razor: The overbrush of unnecessary theoretical dogma is being swept away by an ever-growing recognition of the need for clear observation of behaviorial realities in relation to our modern theories of neurology, cognition, and learning.

The diversity in talent and interest of Erickson's students was a constant source of celebration for him. They ranged from the philosophically oriented J. Beahrs[3] to the modern, psychoanalytically oriented Sidney Rosen[4] to the existentially oriented Len Bergantino.[5] That professionals with widely diverse orientations were consistently attracted to Erickson's work was a testament to both the scope of his own world view as well as to his ability to relate easily and genuinely to the differing views of any truly thoughtful person.

After organizing The American Society of Clinical Hypnosis as an amalgam of physicians, dentists, and psychologists, Erickson wanted other people-helper groups such as social workers, nurses, and even the police, to be trained in the use of hypnosis.

[1] *The Language of Change.* New York: Basic Books, 1978.

[2] M. H. Erickson. *A Teaching Seminar of Milton H. Erickson,* edited by Jeffrey Zeig. New York: Brunner-Mazel, 1980.

[3] J. Beahrs, "Integrating Erickson's Approach." *The American Journal of Clinical Hypnosis,* 1977, *20,* 55–68; and *That Which Is: An Inquiry into the Nature of Energy, Ethics, and Mental Health.* Palo Alto, Calif.: Science and Behavior Books, 1977.

[4] S. Rosen. *My Voice Will Go with You: The Teaching Tales of Milton H. Erickson, M.D.* New York: Norton, 1982.

[5] L. Bergantino. *Psychotherapy, Insight and Style: The Existential Moment.* Boston: Allyn & Bacon, 1981.

He therefore set about personally training representatives from each of these fields. Ironically, many of these carefully trained professionals (such as Dr. Martin Reiser, who wrote *The Handbook of Investigative Hypnosis* [Los Angeles: LEHI, 1980] and has been employed as a psychologist training police in the use of hypnosis) have experienced much professional-political opposition from the established professional organizations that train people only at the doctoral level in the healing professions.

The wider dissemination of Erickson's technique will probably take place through many of the new institutes and organizations that are springing up spontaneously all over the country to train non-doctoral level professionals. There is no official head of all these efforts, but the workshops of The Milton H. Erickson Foundation have Jeffrey K. Zeig, Ph.D., Sherron Peters, Erickson's wife, Elizabeth, and his doctor-daughter, Kristina, as the current directors.[1] Furthermore, The Foundation was organized before Milton's death, and with his active participation. The American Society of Clinical Hypnosis[2] and The Society for Clinical and Experimental Hypnosis[3] remain as the two largest organizations for the training of doctorate-level professionals in the use of hypnosis in this country.

Erickson received many honors throughout his career for his outstanding contributions, but in his later years two awards were especially appreciated: In 1977 he was awarded the Benjamin Franklin Gold Medal by the International Society of Hypnosis, and in July of 1977 a special issue of *The American Journal of Clinical Hypnosis* was published to commemorate his 75th birthday, including a special tribute written by Margaret Mead.

The sage who wanted all his students together sometimes seemed to grow a bit beyond them in the last years of his life, even as he tried to explain it as follows:

[1] Address: 3606 N. 24th Street, Phoenix, Arizona, 85016 (founded by Jeffrey K. Zeig, Ph.D.).

[2] Address: 2400 East Devon, No. 218, Des Plaines, Illinois, 60018.

[3] Address: 129-A Kings Park Dr., Liverpool, New York, 13088.

E: I was in the backyard a year ago in the summertime. I was wondering what far-out experiences I'd like to have. As I puzzled over that, I noticed that I was sitting out in the middle of nowhere. I was an object in space.

K: There you have it: the middle of nowhere.

E: I was just an object in space. Of all the buildings I couldn't see an outline. I couldn't see the chair in which I was sitting; in fact, I couldn't feel it.

R: You spontaneously experienced that vision?

E: It was the most far-out thing I could do!

R: That was the most far-out thing you could do?

E: You can't get more far-out than that!

R: It just happened to you as you were wondering about what you could do?

E: Yes.

R: An unconscious responding?

E: And that was my unconscious' full response.

R: I see; you can't get more far-out than that.

E: What more far-out could happen?

K: You were just floating or just a nothingness?

E: I was just an object and all alone with me was an empty void. No buildings, earth, stars, sun.

K: What emotions did you experience? Did you— curiosity or fear or apprehension?

E: It was one of the most pleasing experiences. What is this? Tremendous comfort. I knew that I was doing something far-out. And I was really doing it! And what greater joy is there than doing what you want to do? Inside the stars, the planets, the beaches. I couldn't feel the weight. I couldn't feel the earth. No matter how much I pushed down my feet, I couldn't feel anything.

R: That sounds like a spontaneous experience of nirvana or samadhi wherein Indian yogis say they experience "the void." You feel that is so?

E: Yes. The far-out experience of negating all reality-related stimuli.

R: That's what the yogis train themselves to do.

E: Yes, just negating the stimuli from the reality objects.

K: You found that pleasurable?

E: I always find when I can do something, it's pleasurable. (pp. 129–130)

Epilogue

Having developed a truly unique grasp of the world by studying and compensating for his own infirmities, Erickson's understanding of human relations was naturally different from that of his colleagues. Thus while he found much in common with his fellow workers, perceptual and communication gaps were ever-present even among those who knew him best. Although he did research on fundamental psychoanalytic concepts with the Freudian theoretician, Lawrence Kubie, and shared views and projects with other eminent thinkers such as Aldous Huxley, Margaret Mead, and Gregory Bateson, Erickson always remained the *sui generis* worker whose extraordinary performance skills remained the centerpiece of his professional identity. None could deny the brilliant and unusual effects he could achieve hypnotically, but few could understand or reproduce his work. This has led to much confusion and misunderstanding about Erickson's contributions and remains as a poignant problem today, even among those who would be his followers: How can the average professional, with all the learned limitations of our average culture, learn to achieve those utterly effective but always unique therapeutic results that were the product of so idiosyncratic an intelligence as Milton H. Erickson?

I believe even this short sketch of Erickson's life provides an important understanding of the source of his genius that is often overlooked by those who seek to emulate the brilliance of his technical accomplishments. Erickson's technique came from his own blood and suffering; his therapeutic originality evolved out of life and death efforts to cope with his own congenital deficiencies and crippling physical illnesses. I believe this is the true source of his effectiveness as a therapist: patients could sense on many levels that Erickson's therapeutic skill came from genuine personal experience and knowledge. He truly was the wounded physician who through healing himself had learned how to heal others. The same is true for all of us who experience a genuine calling to the healing professions. We are all wounded in one way or another. Our always partial success in healing our own wounds leads us to our calling to explore with others further means of coping and extending the possibilities of our mutually human condition.

Patients rightly resent it when they feel they are being manipulated by the "empty technique" employed by an operator who has no personal connection and knowledge of the shared sources of problems and illness within all of us. Such operators attempt to use technique as a means of power and prestige to control others. But of course the patient's unconscious can pick up the shallowness of this empty charade, and nothing really changes; "resistances" only become manifest. Even if a symptom is changed, there still has been no deepening association with the inner sources of illness and creativity that are the true quest of all healing work.

It is to this end that this brief overview of Erickson's life and these volumes of his seminars, workshops, and lectures are dedicated: How can each of us create a more effective relationship with the sources and problems of our own uniqueness? How can we refine these skills in helping others cope with the dilemmas of our mutually human condition?

PART I

UTILIZING UNCONSCIOUS
PROCESSES IN HYPNOSIS*

The Course of Scientific and Medical History:
From Nonsense and Superstition to Fact

The topics I want to talk about concern hypnosis in general, but there are some opening remarks that I want to make first. A long time ago in medical history there was a man named [Edward] Jenner who observed certain things. Among his observations was the discovery that if a milkmaid got cow pox then she was vaccinated against small pox. And Jenner promolgated that horrible idea of impurifying human blood by contaminating it with cow pox. And if you go through some of the papers written on the subject of vaccination long ago, you will discover that when that hideous art of vaccination was practiced, otherwise nice, young men and women would develop hooves and horns and would bellow like cattle! [Laughter] That's one of the scientific discoveries of medicine by some of the proponents of these rash developments.

And then, you know, in the early days of transfusion scientific papers were written against it by various learned people who warned that if you were not careful, that if you did not really understand, that if you transfused female blood into a man—well, let's take it the other way: if you gave masculine blood to a female, she—well, let's go back to the first one! [Laughter] I think you're beginning to get the idea that young men would grow breasts, and while it was never really proved that a girl could get pregnant from masculine blood there was

*Lecture given in San Francisco, California, 1961

some hint that girls would develop beards, and their voices would deepen, and all that sort of nonsense. But those papers were written up by the authors with absolute belief in the scientific validity of the ideas expressed therein. And while one can credit the integrity of the authors of those papers, one wonders about their scientific knowledge at that time.

And one of the most delightful ideas I ever read about was expressed in a series of papers by a Massachusetts physician. His message was that if anybody, just *anybody,* were foolish enough to ride on that new-fangled contraption called the railroad, and if the train one were riding in exceeded the horrible speed of 15 m.p.h., then it would result in the suffocation of the person who faced into that horrible wind. So he advocated that the railroad management be compelled to put up shelters over the seats and to have all the seats face backwards in order to prevent the suffocation of people. Now I read a whole series of such papers by that physician—I wonder where he was when the wind blew in Massachusetts. He didn't add that as a footnote, but I was curious about it! [Laughter]

And then not so awfully long ago there were any number of people—intelligent, competent, capable people—who gladly explained to Henry Ford that the horse was here to stay. And Henry Ford was so stupid that he wouldn't listen to them, he just wouldn't listen. "But the horse is here to stay!" they all cried. And there was a lot of comment on that.

And then, you know, the Wright brothers really should have had their heads examined because they thought a machine heavier than air could fly; and there were innumerable mathematical formulae devised to prove conclusively that machines heavier than air could not fly.

When heart surgery was first developed, [the same sort of nonsensical ideas prefaced its acceptance]. And then, quite some time ago, there was that rather undesirable person in Wisconsin who advocated the setting up of private clinics for the treatment of venereal disease. For this he was promptly kicked out of all medical societies because, the reason went, if you set up private clinics for the treatment of venereal disease you will really be promoting its spread, for no one would go into such a clinic except for the purposes of purely private gain.

And, I think it was in 1929 that Surgeon General [Thomas] Parran dared to give an interview to the newspapers in which he mentioned the names of two types of venereal disease. And there was much to-do and much condemnation of Surgeon General Parran for daring to give those words to the newspaper where the eyes of innocent young readers would be subjected to them. And yet the result of his action was a tremendous decrease in the incidence of syphilis of the brain in mental hospitals. But Surgeon General Parran was roundly condemned, and those condemnations came from the West Coast to the East Coast, from churches, from medical societies, from everywhere.

And then that man from Wisconsin who had advocated private clinics for the treatment of venereal disease was kicked out of his county medical society, out of the state medical society, and he was denied membership in the American Medical Association. Then in 1956 he was admitted to honorary membership in the AMA, but by that time he just didn't care.

When Psychoanalysis was first introduced to the United States there were only two courses open for the analyst and for the analysand. The analysand would become promiscuous—there was no doubt at all about that; and the analyst—he himself would wind up in the state hospital, because that's what Psychoanalysis did to people. And I listened to a great deal of criticism of Psychoanalysis in the teens and in the twenties, and I can remember the President of the American Neurological Association, whose prime boast was that he had never been west of the Hudson River; and he had lots and lots to say in the denunciation of Psychoanalysis.

Then, not so very long ago I read some very, very learned articles which explained that supersonic speed would result in the molecular disintegration of the plane and of the pilot. And I thought that would be a fascinating experience for any pilot and for any plane! [Laughter] And I wondered when it had happened, and I wondered how the writer of that paper really knew.

Now I've mentioned all these stories because the course of human understanding, the course of medical science, has been marked by that sort of thing. And now shall we pause a moment in honor of Harold Rosen? [Much laughter; audience breaks into applause.] *

Management of Parents by Children: A Two-Year-Old's Indirect Hypnotic Technique

Now what I would like to say concerns the matter of interpersonal communication which constitutes what hypnosis is really about. And I'd like to impress upon you the importance of this matter of human intercommunication. And I'm going to give you a case history to illustrate my point.

I was waiting for a plane in Midway Airport in Chicago a while back when a young mother I judged to be about 28 years old came in with her toddling two-year-old. They sat down on the bench near me—it was a long bench. Now the two-year-old was a little bit irritable. Mother was tired and she had a newspaper; she spread it open and began reading it. And the two-year-old got up and walked the length of the bench. I, having nothing else to do except to wait for my plane, watched that two-year-old. And when the two-year-old reached the end of the bench she looked at that toy counter over there, turned and looked at mother, saw that mother was reading, turned and looked back at the toy counter; now she just looked and looked, and after what appeared to be much thought and reflection, went back beside mother and jumped up and down. Mother said, "Be quiet!", so the child got down on the floor and started running around. Mother hauled the child back to the bench and said, "Sit still!" The child got up and raced up and down, looked at the toy counter, looked at mother, raced up and down. Mother said, "Stop it! Sit down! Lie down! Go to sleep! Rest! Quit annoying me!" (You know, mothers sometimes do that!)

Editors' Note: This is an example of Erickson's humor. Harold Rosen was a medical colleague who had recently been raising a great deal of controversy over his view of hypnosis as dangerous. The audience was very much aware that Erickson held the opposite viewpoint.

Well, the child would obediently lie down for a few seconds, then spring up, go down and see if that toy were still there, look at mother, and then start racing. Finally mother said, "If you want some exercise, I'll give it to you!" So the child took mother by the hand, walked her clear around on that side, and just by accident they stopped at the toy counter. Mother looked and said, "Maybe there is something here that will make you behave"! [Much laughter] I think that was one of the most beautiful examples of indirect hypnotic technique I have ever witnessed.

Now, who taught that child that sort of technique? How did the child know? The child is a rather primitive being; it's rather responsive to the things that adults do to it. And so that two-year-old, with all the wisdom of its infancy uncomplicated by the false learnings that society and convention force upon us, reacted to its own understanding: "I want that toy; Mother often says no; maybe the best thing to do is to annoy her and give her a chance to quiet me down." [Laughter] I don't think the child thought all that out very clearly, but I watched the entire episode wondering just exactly how that child was going to get the toy. I thought—but then I'm an adult—that the child would simply take mother and lead her right over. But the child was a lot brighter than I was—she knew the right technique!*

The Unconscious Mind in Hypnosis: Utilizing a Vast Reservoir of Learning

All of you think that when you work with hypnosis you need to devise it and work with it as a means of communicating this or that idea to the patient. I think you ought to recognize that the unconscious of the human being is a rather comprehending thing. There is a whole biological history behind the separation of the unconscious mind—a convenient concept, because it does describe a certain type of behavior. The biological history of the human race discloses that a great deal of human behavior never comes to conscious awareness, yet it is employed extensively to

*Editors' Note: This story is repeated in Part IV.

govern people. I don't think that little two-year-old had ever figured out in conscious terms how to manage mother, but that child certainly did know how to manage mother.

I think that all of us ought to recognize that there are a tremendous number of things that we first learn on a conscious level in order to do them more adequately and effortlessly. Now those of you who heard me mention this example earlier will forgive my repetition. Take the person who is learning to drive a car: "Now, let's see. . . . I put my left foot on the clutch. . . . I put my right foot on the accelerator. . . . I hold the steering wheel this way. . . . Oh, but I'd better have the right hand a little bit lower than the left—or is it the other way around! And now, I can start the car." And that person goes through this laborious, conscious procedure of analyzing his behavior until one day he gets into his car and drives clear across town in traffic, all the while talking to a delightful friend. And he is so surprised when he turns into the right driveway, because he didn't even know that he had been on the other side of town. He aparently had driven safely since he didn't receive any traffic tickets; yet he couldn't remember having passed this section of town, because he was so absorbed. In some way he had been driving his car at an unconscious level while directing his conscious attention to the conversation.

Everybody knows how to tie a shoestring until you ask them how they did it, and then they don't seem to know very much about it. And practically any man can tie a bow tie on himself until you ask him, "Now just which hand moves first?" And, of course, you know that delightful poem by Ogden Nash that I like to misquote: there is that centipede that is getting along so well until someone asks it, "Which foot comes after which?", and now that poor centipede is lying in a ditch! [Laughter]

I talked to a student of words and semantics the other day who said, "You know, if you repeat a word a half dozen times you begin to wonder how that word came to mean anything at all; you come to wonder why that word is so fitting for its object." And that is true, because we unconsciously sort out from our lifetime of experiences the things that we keep as conscious understandings, and then we put into the unconscious

66

mind a tremendous number of other understandings. I think that when you use hypnosis in the handling of patients and in the treatment of various conditions you ought to rely upon that vast reservoir of learning that the unconscious mind has. We all know that we can go to a suspenseful movie and lose a headache without ever getting an intravenous injection, without swallowing a drug, without altering the sensory nerves in any way. And how does a suspenseful movie counteract a headache?—but it does happen. By what sort of processes? By the establishment of trains of thought, trains of associations, and by the stimulation of other forms of activity. And why would you use hypnosis except to achieve the same sort of purpose.

Psychopathology as an Index of Reverse Potentials: The Untutored Boy

I can think of the case of a 15-year-old boy who came from a rural community, had had very little contact with the external world, had gone to school only through the sixth grade, and who worked on his father's farm. When he was admitted to the state hospital it was my task to examine him and interview him. And I was utterly fascinated when I asked him to draw a picture of a man. He drew a very nice picture of a man, and I showed it to the two psychologists of the hospital, as well as to several psychiatrists. One of the psychologists went into his office, unlocked a desk drawer, and brought out that volume of Princehorn. Princehorn was a German writer who had collected the drawings of psychotics. We matched my patient's picture of a man against the one that Princehorn had reproduced in his book and found that the measurements were essentially the same. There was a certain similarity between the peculiar drawing of Princehorn's psychotic patient and that of my psychotic patient. One almost thought my patient's drawing was a copy of the other one. And I do know that that one copy of Princehorn was the only copy known to exist in the state of Massachusetts at the time—because, you see, it's a rather rare volume.

Then in taking the young man's mental history I discovered

one of the most utterly involved systems of psychopathology— of delusions, hallucinations, and symbolism—that I had ever seen. It would have taken any well-trained psychiatrist years and years to unravel. Now, just how did an untutored, 15-year-old boy manage to devise such an elaborate delusional system? I mention this story because you ought to bear in mind that sort of thing when you work with a patient: *you ought to expect your patient to be willing to devise elaborate things of a good character as well as of a bad character.* And you can use hypnosis to motivate people in the working for their own welfare and benefit.*

The Rapid Resolution of an Acute Obsessional Phobia: The Fortieth Birthday Phobia

Now I want to cite another case. The man I am thinking of had a birthday on August the 3rd of this year when he turned forty years old. I took a rather extensive history of him. It seems that in his teens he had a tendency to look upon the age of forty as the time when he'd be an old man; a time when his head would be thrust forward, his shoulders would be rounded forward, and he'd be walking with a stoop, completely uninterested in any of the delightful things in life. And on a particular occasion in his early twenties he happened to feel sorry for some poor old duffer who was forty years old—my word, how old can a person get! And then again in his later twenties he had another occasion to feel sorry for an aged forty-year-old. Then the matter rather dropped out of his thinking. He was a professional man, not from the field of medicine, but from another professional field. He enjoyed his work, he enjoyed his associates, he enjoyed his hobbies; he enjoyed being elected president of this particular group, president of that particular group, being chairman of this committee and of that committee. He had but one bitter disappointment in his life: He and his wife had no children.

Editors' Note: This story is repeated in Part III, with slightly different perspectives.

And then on July 17th of this year he attended a party where everything went very, very nicely. There was a very nice chicken dinner and salad, which he ate, and then about three o'clock that morning he developed a terrific stomach ache. He got horribly frightened, and with some difficulty managed to get out of that rather lonesome part of the country and back to civilization. And the first doctor he called upon for a check-up was on vacation, so he was hurriedly taken to another hospital and hospitalized immediately.

The doctor came in and said to my patient: "You are sweating too much; your respiration is bad; I'm going to run a heart examination (an EKG) on you." There were about six frames taken—that is a picture about so long—and then the machine broke down and the doctor said: "Well, there's just enough here to indicate that we ought to go carefully. But I'm going to refer you to Dr. X because I start my vacation tomorrow. [Laughter]

So Dr. X looked over the case and said, "We'll have to get an EKG. This has got to be looked into. But I really can't take charge of your case because I'm leaving on vacation. I've got a very nice young assistant coming in, and I'm sure he will be quite able to take care of you." So my patient went to the young assistant who said, "Now let's really work up this case." [Laughter] And they did work up his case. They counted his toes and his toenails, his fingers and his fingernails, just to make sure he had a full supply of everything. They really did a most comprehensive examination. And the man lay there gasping, wondering, "What's wrong!" He didn't know that they were doing a comprehensive examination. After the assistant got this man's case all worked up, his mother developed a cardiac condition and so he [the assistant] flew East. [Laughter] My patient was then sent to someone else. It took four long months for him to finally receive a diagnosis: "There's absolutely nothing wrong with your heart, your lungs, your liver. All you had was an acute colonic spasm—nothing more. You've got nothing at all to worry about."

But the man came to me and said: "But I *do* have something to worry about. Every time I hear a sound I wonder if I'm going batty. I went through all that anxiety and all that difficulty. I think I've got an iatrogenic psychosis caused by the doctor!"

Now what had this man done? He couldn't tolerate the thought of anything being wrong with his body; he couldn't tolerate the thought of heart disease; so he translated his fear of physical illness into a multitude of psychological fears and anxieties.

In the office with me he said: "I'm afraid you're going to try to reassure me. I want you to put me in a trance; I want you to correct my ideas; I've been to three men already in the hope of being put in a trance—because I really want to be told to forget these types of ideas: 'Is that a voice over here I'm hearing? Or is that a voice over there I'm hearing?' I want to forget that sort of acute obsessional fear that I have."

But when I tried to induce a trance in the man—because he demanded that I try—he just straightened up and looked at me and said, "I wish I could cooperate with you, but every time you say something I become increasingly alert." And that's why I want to mention this particular story: You must recognize that whatever your patient brings to you constitutes a legitimate part of his condition. Just as the patient may be allergic to aspirin, the patient may be allergic to a drug, and you ought to respect that. Some patients can't stand adhesive on their skin; others can't tolerate iodine without getting a severe rash or burn as a result. Similarly, you ought to respect whatever intolerances patients have toward certain ideas.

Inducing a Hyper-alert Trance by the Fixation of Attention

To get back to the case, I asked my patient to please let me handle the case as a psychiatrist. Never mind the fact that I had some experience in hypnosis, let me handle it as a psychiatrist. And would he please look at the clock there and notice the edge of it; would he please listen to the ticking of the clock and hear it plainly. And bear in mind that he could stay awake, and that his awareness of the sight of the clock, of the ticking of the clock, of the fact that I had his wife sitting beside him, could prove to him that he was wide awake; that he was not going into a trance; that I was not going to overcome him in some way and force him to develop the amnesia that he requested and resisted—because he *did* want an amnesia and he *didn't* want an amnesia.

Now, by fixating his gaze on the sight of the clock, by fixating his hearing on the tick of the clock, by fixating his awareness of his position in the office by the presence of his wife sitting beside him, I was then able to take a comprehensive history of him. He was able to talk to me about his past and he was able to discuss it in a sympathetic way. He could understand how seriously affected he had been by one, particular, circumscribed idea. He understood that he had had a tremendous fear of that birthday of his coming up on the 3rd of August; and it is July 17th at the party, and on August 3rd he would be forty years old—over the hill, really gone, nothing to ever look forward to in life. He had all that teenage, childhood, childish thinking about the remote age of forty.

Now I handled his particular situation not by telling him to relax, not by telling him to go into a trance, not by telling him to feel comfortable and at ease. Instead, I fixated him visually and auditorily on the clock, and I fixated him interpersonally on the position of his wife beside him. And in that utterly completely secure position—where he could see the clock plainly, where he could hear the clock plainly, where he could glance out of his peripheral vision to see his wife plainly—in that position he could give all his attention to an orderly discussion and thinking through of his problem.

Now, previous to the onset of that colonic spasm the man had been very happy and well adjusted. Illness can come on all of a sudden; one can make a massive response all at once to a particular thing. I do not think we should assume that in every such instance we need to presuppose or propound some long, drawn-out causation and a long, drawn-out therapeutic process. You see, *if illness can occur suddenly, then therapy can occur quite as suddenly.*

I saw this patient a total of six hours—three interviews, each two hours long. The man has returned to his work and he is free of his obsessional, fearful ideas. And he can talk about all those anxieties and hallucinations—about all the auditory, visual, tactile, gustatory, olfactory hallucinations. He had such a great wealth of psychopathology that didn't really fit together. He'll be back to see me next month, and he intends to write a letter each week simply because he thinks I'm a nice person to write to. I have no particular worries or fears about him because I have a feeling that he will get along very, very satisfactorily.

Sudden "Spontaneous" Life Transformations: Healing Can Be as Rapid as Illness

I have seen a great wealth of things happen in my experience. I can think of that 25-year-old man who had served time in prison, who had been drunk regularly, who had committed every offense imaginable, who was a completely undesirable citizen. I saw that man condemned thoroughly by competent members of society who were utterly despairing of him; and I also saw that young man walk down a street, unsuspectingly encounter a very charming bit of flotsam, and within the next year become a happily married, solid, substantial citizen. And that very charming bit of fluff did not have a single brain cell, except the kind that made that man want to do all the good things in the world.

I can think of a patient I encountered in Phoenix. She was in her 25th year and she had been a professional for some ten years. She gave me a very elaborate account of places in Detroit; she knew all the gossip about the city of Detroit, and she named all the streets in correct fashion; she'd been in Chicago and in New York; she knew the correct name for the hotel; she knew the superintendent's name. I had no doubt about the validity of her story. Then she told me about how she had come out of a grocery store one day with a pie, because she maintained her own apartment—she made her living in her apartment—and encountered a young man. For some reason he looked like a very nice citizen to her, and she decided right then and there that she was going to marry him. It was utterly charming to listen to her account of her decision right then and there. She promptly moved to another neighborhood and changed her name. She had noted the license number on her young man's car; she had found out what church he was going to; she had managed to hunt him up. And now she has been happily married to him for about five years. She came to see me about what a stepmother should do to promote the love affair of her stepson whom she had acquired when she married that young widower.

Now just exactly what was the therapeutic process that took place in that girl in that particular situation? Was she just romanticizing? I don't think so. She was straightforward and frank with me; she told me her history because she thought that perhaps my understanding of her history would give me an understanding of her as a human personality. And she was very definitely concerned about "giving my son [the proper guidance]." You see, she preferred to call him "my son," although she made certain that I understood he was really her stepson. She was concerned and interested and delighted to have the opportunity of being a normal woman, living a normal life, free from all of that peculiar stress and strain of ten years of professional life in Chicago, in Detroit, in New York, in various other places.

Now, when these casual, incidental influences and occurrences in life—completely unplanned and uncalculated—manage to transform a person so very, very thoroughly and so very, very suddenly, it signifies that there was a certain readiness for change in that person. But what about the patient who comes to you who wants therapy. And what kind of therapy does he really want from you? Does he want a complete understanding of himself, or does he want to use you to achieve certain unrecognized goals and purposes?

Applying "Child Psychology" (the *Child's* Psychology) in the Treatment of Adult Patients: The Case of the Hopeless Student

I have a most delightful patient who came to me last May to tell me about his future academic plans, wishes, and desires. And as I listened to him last May I wanted to explain to him (and finally I did explain to him) that the best thing for him to do would be to notify the medical school that he didn't want to enroll as a freshman medic. Why be accepted as a student, and then when medical school opens, fail to attend? And he assured me over and over again that he was going to enroll as a freshman medic. I knew that he wasn't going to attend, because he lacked five hours' work to get his BA degree. He'd been accepted by the medical school on the condition that he would have earned his BA degree by the time he enrolled for the first semester.

Now, he needed only five hours of work; he had nothing to do the entire month of June; nothing to do the entire month of July; and he was a very brilliant, very capable, utterly charming chap. And I pointed out to him, "You know, you ought to plan to have that five hours of scholastic work done by Saturday. Suppose you tell me about your completion of it on Monday." Monday came and he did not have the work completed, but he said he would have it done by the next Saturday. My statement was, "Suppose you tell me about it a week from today on Monday; suppose you tell me about it on the last day in June. . . . on the 7th day of July. . . . on the 15th day of July. . . . the 31st of July. . . . on August the 1st. . . . on August the 23rd. . . . on September the 1st."

The last day before he could get credit from the registrar and receive his BA degree he finished that five hours of course work. Then he went to the registrar, but he arrived one hour after the office closed! And that was the last day he could file the information. So he'll get his BA degree next January. Entrance to medical school is contingent upon that degree. Why would he do that sort of thing? When he came to me I knew what he was going to do, but there was no way that I could influence him hypnotically or otherwise. He wanted to do it that way. He introduced me to the girl he was going to marry. I looked at the girl—she was an awfully nice girl—and I knew that he was going to break that engagement; but he didn't know it. He became converted to another religious faith; he's now in the process of discovering that he's going to be *un*converted. [Laughter] This past week he applied for admission to another medical school; he was already enrolled to take postgraduate work, and it seems he will be going to that medical school with a record of failing grades in his postgraduate work! Now, can hypnosis help him? Can psychiatry help him? Can psychotherapy help him? He needs a tremendous amount of help. He is intelligent; he is capable. As a therapist, you would need to have a willingness to suggest to him the importance of facing things, of understanding things, but without trying to crowd him. You would have to use hypnosis gently, carefully, and indirectly. You couldn't do very much for this patient, but bear in mind that that two-year-old child maneuvered her mother around to the toy counter in the most absolutely beautiful fashion. I think you have to look upon the handling of adult patients in the same sort of fashion. I wish I had as much skill with this college student as that two-year-old had with her mother. But I haven't!

Utilizing the Unconscious in Hypnosis to Communicate Ideas and Activate Latent Potentialities

I've given you these different cases because I want to impress upon you that the unconscious knows a tremendous amount. You don't have to explain too much, you don't have to argue too much; you do have to recognize the personality forces involved, and you do have to recognize the gentleness and effectiveness with which you can give ideas so that patients will incorporate them. The most I can do for this young man is to get him to accept the idea that perhaps he had better see me somewhere around once every three weeks. I wanted to see him more often, but in looking him over I saw the set of that jaw, I saw the narrowing of his eyes, so I weakened to two weeks, I weakened to three weeks. He thinks I'm a rather intelligent and capable person, because he had a very agreeable expression on his face when he left. And so I'm seeing him about every three weeks. Maybe sooner or later I can get across to him the idea that we ought to take up a number of other factors that are disturbing his successful adjustment as a competent personality. You see, you have to respect the patient, and you have to bear in mind that his unconscious takes a certain attitude toward the total personality; you've got to deal with that, and you've got to realize that your purpose in using hypnosis is not to effect magic. *Your purpose in using hypnosis is to communicate ideas and understandings and to get the patient to utilize the competencies that exist within him at both a psychological level and a physiological level.*

That patient of mine who had the history of the colonic spasm now has the attitude that "I just hope I get another colonic spasm, and I'm going to lie down and I'm going to tell my colon that it's a darn nice thing to own, and I couldn't get along without it." [Laughter] In other words, he has a totally different perspective from his original one of fear and anxiety. His new attitude has a touch of meanness in it—like the child. You've seen the little child who is so pleased with being the self and who conveys that so nicely. And I think this particular patient is going to have that completely happy, simple, childish contentment with the physical self: "I am me, and I'm glad I'm me; and now what can I do with the me that I have." And when you can convey that sort of understanding to a patient then you will have enlisted his physiological cooperation as well as his psychological cooperation. But I think I've talked long enough, and thanks very much for listening. If you have any questions I shall be delighted to try to answer them.

DEMONSTRATION: TRANCE IN THERAPY AND IN EVERYDAY LIFE

Response Attentiveness and the Selection of Subjects for Hypnotic Demonstration

E: Well, let's see. Who shall I select as a subject? I've seen some very interesting faces around here tonight. I've seen some faces where, as I glanced about the room with my hand up, I saw that thought travel across: "I wonder if he's going to pick on me!" [Laughter] Now why shouldn't I? Those were pretty faces I saw that thought go over!

Rossi (R): Although Erickson appears to be very casual in the selection of subjects from the audience at this point, he has, in fact, already developed a good rapport—both with the audience in general and with specific individuals in particular—during the previous lecture. While lecturing he has been looking for those members of the audience who give evidence of good response attentiveness; that is, he looks for those individuals who are responding with great absorption to his talk and person. High response attentiveness is shown when individuals are so absorbed in receiving everything the lecturer is saying that their bodies become quiet and motionless, they stare at the speaker with dilated pupils and slack facial expressions, and they tend to nod their heads slowly in the affirmative. Erickson describes more about this to the audience below.

These are the "interesting faces" to Erickson. He then shares his observations about how he reads in their "pretty" faces the thought, "I wonder if he is going to pick me." Of course the audience responds with laughter because he is so correct in reading their body language. With all this he is reinforcing the good mood of positive expectation that he developed during his lecture about the wonderful, indirect, rapid, healing outcomes that can occur through the person's unconscious in hypnosis. Who wouldn't want to experience such a marvelous process? We can thus look upon his entire lecture as an indirect hypnotic approach to priming and facilitating each individual's unconscious trance potentials for the interesting hypnotic demonstration that is now to take place.

Group Support in Hypnotic Work

E: You know, I'm color blind, and I don't know whether that's a green sweater or a blue blouse, but it is a flat collar, I think! [Laughter] Do you mind coming? Would you come over to my left? Will you step closer? Have you ever been in a trance before?

Subject (S): No, I don't think so.

E: But you do work for Dr. Reed, he says? You're not going to advertise that after *this,* are you! [Laughter] Have you seen him do hypnosis?

S: Yes.

E: Are you interested in going into a trance?

S: [Pause] Yes [said hesitantly and with a nervous chuckle].

E: You could be more enthusiastic! But now if you will look somewhat to your left you'll see a blue-dressed girl. I think she ought to come up here too, don't you?

S: Oh, yes!

E: Come on, Mary. Now, shall I give any discussion of why I am doing it this way? [Yeses from the audience] Not because it makes it more difficult for me.

R: Erickson now casually uses his own colorblindness to disarm and humorously reassure his shy subject. By selecting another woman, Mary, as a second subject, he further reassures the first subject and gives her a model (Mary) of how to behave hypnotically.

Erickson frequently used his own infirmities and stories about growth and healing in his family or in other patients to activate similar healing processes in his subjects. While these healing stories can be regarded as metaphorical, it is important to recognize that Erickson usually did not make them up—his examples and stories were true.* This is in great contrast to some students who claim to be using Ericksonian approaches when they confabulate what they hope will be a therapeutic metaphor.

In the above lecture Erickson evidences great respect for

Editors' Note: An exception would be Erickson's use of pseudoscientific explanations for intellectually naive subjects who needed a concrete image of healing they could understand from their own life perspective.

the patient's own unconscious and its potentials to effect the therapeutic process. I believe that the great potency of Erickson's healing stories was at least partly due to the absolute conviction with which they were presented—having been genuinely experienced in a deep and moving way by Erickson himself.

Much recent research on vocal stress patterns as well as body language patterns points to our unconscious capacity to separate truth from falsehood, even when the conscious mind apparently accepts the falsehood. When this happens, further conflicts are set up within the individual, who is now split between believing and not believing. In the therapy setting, patients already come in with enough doubt. If a therapist then makes up metaphors which he himself does not believe, stress of some sort would probably infiltrate his vocal and behavioral patterns. These stress patterns would then be received by the patient as ambiguous messages that could only serve to reduce whatever credibility the therapist's words might have had on an unconscious level within the patient. Indeed, human truth pierces us in a way that confabulated metaphor can only parody.

Questions, Doubt, Confusion, and Vocal Cues in Hypnotic Induction

E: Mary, have you ever been in a trance before?

Mary (M): I don't think so.

E: You don't think so. And you're not going to think so. [Voice softens considerably] Alright, and now— [pause]

R: Here Erickson casually introduces a number of his indirect hypnotic approaches with these few remarks. First, questioning about any previous trance experience tends to reactivate trance memories and so indirectly facilitates the current initiation of a similar condition.

Next, Erickson's response of "You don't think so" to

Mary's answer, "I don't think so," may contain an important implication of doubt. There is often a vast gulf between how we view our own subjective experiences and how others view them. Most of us are in ongoing states, conscious or unconscious, of doubt, confusion and conflict with others about these differing points of view. With that one seemingly casual response, "You don't think so," Erickson is evoking and utilizing this vast reservoir of inner doubt and confusion to depotentiate Mary's current mental sets so that an altered state may be facilitated.

Erickson's next sentence, "And you're not going to think so," is even more ambiguous: while seeming to agree with Mary's point of view, there is at the same time a confusing implication in it such that she cannot reject it. Erickson may be setting up a double bind which he will use later to ratify the trance experience. If, for example, Mary later denies that she experienced trance, Erickson can precipitate a conscious-unconscious double bind by casually questioning, "And you really don't *think* you did, did you?" In an atmosphere where doubt and confusion are already brewing, this question would effectively depotentiate the conscious mind's confidence in its assessment of its own experience.

Notice also the softening of Erickson's voice as he makes this statement. This softening of the voice was Erickson's way of utilizing a cue familiar to most of us from earliest childhood when mother softened her voice while rocking us to sleep. Voices also seem to soften and grow dim in everyday life when we are self-absorbed, and right before we fall asleep.

Hand Levitation with a Time Double Bind and "Not Knowing" Facilitating Hypnotic Induction

[Although it is not obvious from the tape, Dr. David Cheek who was present in the audience, confirmed that Erickson began a typical hand levitation approach to trance at about this point.]

M: I don't know whether you're shaking or I'm shaking!
[Laughter]

E: Are you concerned about that shaking or that tremulousness?

M: Yes, because I think [remainder of sentence lost in recording].

E: But you don't need to be worried about it.

M: No.

E: And when do you think your eyes will close?

M: I don't know.

E: Before or after your hand touches your face?

M: I don't know.

R: Erickson facilitates a hand levitation by gently providing very light multiple touches on Mary's wrist and arm that confuse her conscious mind but direct her unconscious mind to lift.* (Polio residuals often left Erickson with a tremor in his right hand.) Once the hand and arm are levitating in a seemingly autonomous manner, the next step is to facilitate eye closure. Erickson does this with a double binding question, "When do you think *your eyes will close*. . . . before or after *your hand touches your face?*" He is actually giving two strongly directive suggestions in an indirect manner so that they reinforce each other: (1) *your eyes will close* (it's only a matter of time, before or after), and (2) *your hand will touch your face.* The strongly directive orientation of these suggestions is

*See *Experiencing Hypnosis* for extensive discussion of and exercises for this approach.

disguised by the way Erickson is apparently allowing Mary to have some choice about it. (Erickson's colleague, the psychoanalyst Lawrence Kubie, called it "illusory choice.")

Already within this section Mary's ego consciousness is depotentiated to the point where she says "I don't know" at least three times. This *not knowing* facilitates trance and a receptivity to Erickson by simple default.

Direct Suggestions for Eye Closure and Trance Deepening

E: And that blinking. [Pause, very soft] Close your eyes now. That's right. [Long pause] And close your eyes. [Pause] And what I would like to have you do, Mary, is go deeper and deeper in the trance, and [addressing other subject] I would like to have you go deeper and deeper in the trance.

Selecting Hypnotic Subjects via Observation: "Looking Around the Room"

Now, of course that puts both of these young ladies very much on the spot. It makes it very difficult for them. But then you have patients come into your office who are anxious and fearful and uncertain and undecided, and you have to deal with them. My purpose in conducting the demonstration in this way is to let you know that you can, by simply meeting patients and attending to them, give them opportunities to respond. And by fixating their gaze and their attention, you can meet their anxieties; and you don't need to be frightened or distressed by the fact that you do have a tremor of your own hand as a result of fatigue and the residuals of polio, and you can allow patients to interpret it as part of their own behavior.

And now Mary is going deeper and deeper in the trance. I saw her during the cocktail hour, and I was very much impressed by Mary. And I was also very much impressed by Joan [the other subject, named for the first time] as she sat up there. You know, I like to look around a room, because as you look around a room you see the people who listen to others, who try to understand, who want to get a new idea or a new understanding. They are the people who let you complete what you are saying, present their own ideas, and then again listen to yours. And I watched Mary out there in the other room, and I was very much impressed by that nice, attentive responsiveness to the people she was talking to and listening to. And watching Joan up there at the table, speaking to others and listening to others, I thought what an utterly charming personality she was in her capacity to listen, to look, to see, to respond.

And in the audience there happens to be someone else who impressed me in that same way some time ago, and it was so delightful the first time I saw that particular person because of that very delightful responsiveness capacity. And the years that have passed since I met that person have justified me in that feeling of regard and respect and admiration.

Building Hypnotic Phenomena
Bit by Bit

Now, when you get one bit of hypnotic phenomenon, no matter how small it is, there should be an earnest respect for it on your part because it is the foundation for still more and more hypnotic phenomena. And you see Mary is standing there and she is showing a certain amount of catalepsy, and she is showing a tremendous loss of self-consciousness. She hasn't lost all the quivering of her eyes, and I don't know that she ever will lose it because I don't know enough about her. All I know is that there is a certain amount of relaxation in her legs, in her body; but there's a certain amount of body balance there that is perfectly remarkable.

Trance Awakening after Suggestions
for Further Trance Phenomena

E: I know that Joan is standing here very, very comfortably. And I'll make use of these phenomena to establish various other ones. But why shouldn't I ask Mary to take a deep breath? And you can take a deep breath, Mary. And then I'd like to have you rouse up and feel at ease and comfortable.

[Pause] And take all the time you need. Take a deep breath and rouse up feeling so comfortable, Mary. [Very long pause of 20 seconds or so] Wider and wider awake, Mary.

Ratifying Trance and Indirect Permission to Lapse Back into a Relaxed Trance

E: That's it. Quite a job waking up, isn't it? Do you remember telling me out in the cocktail room that you'd never been in a trance?

M: Yes.

E: What do you think about your ability?

M: I still don't know. [Laughter]

E: You still don't know?

M: I know I'm relaxed, but I couldn't answer you.

E: You couldn't answer me?

M: No, you asked me if I had ever been in a trance and I said I didn't think I had.

E: Do you think you have tonight?

M: Do I think . . . ?

E: Do you think you're in a trance right now?

M: Possibly . . . yes . . . I'm relaxed. I thought I'd be self-conscious up here in front of everyone, and I'm not too.

E: Isn't that nice? [Laughter] They're [audience members] really not bad to look at, are they?

M: No . . . they're lovely!

R: With his initial remark of "That's it" followed by the question of "Quite a job waking up, wasn't it?", Erickson is beginning the important process of trance ratification. On awakening from trance, patients typically do not know whether or not they have experienced an altered state. Erickson's question focuses the subject's attention inwardly and implies she will find evidence for recognizing her altered state.

It is usually difficult for beginning students of hypnosis to come to a full realization of the extent to which the conscious mind does not recognize when it is experiencing an altered state. Our extroverted culture asks us nothing about our inner states: We normally need let others know only if we are awake or asleep. So ignorant are we of ourselves that we do not even recognize the obvious stresses and bodily responses by which we create our own psychosomatic ills. Even how to relax, a normal psychophysiological function that takes place naturally every 90 to 120 minutes* is lost to most of us.

Further ratification of trance now takes place via audience laughter when Mary again says she does not know. She confesses her not knowing in three successive answers to Erickson's three queries, finally admits that she is relaxed, and is in fact so lacking in self-consciousness in front of the audience that she then lapses back into trance—if, indeed, she ever really woke up. Erickson immediately reinforces her lapsing back into trance with his indirect, casual remark, "Isn't that nice?" Now Mary is in trance with her eyes open and talking—agreeing with Erickson's suggestion that the audience is "really not bad to look at."

---

*Editors' Note: For discussions of the ultradian cycle, see J. Hiatt and D. Kripke, "Ultradian Rhythms in Waking Gastric Activity," *Psychosomatic Medicine,* 1975, *37,* pp. 330-325; *Experiencing Hypnosis;* and "Hypnotist Describes Natural Rhythm of Trance Readiness," *Brain/Mind Bulletin,* Vol. 6, No. 7, March 30, 1981; E. Rossi, "Hypnosis and Ultradian Cycles: A New State(s) Theory of Hypnosis?", *The American Journal of Clinical Hypnosis,* 1982, *25,* 21-32.

Catalepsy: Distinguishing Between Real and Fake Trance with Tactile Cues

E: Now why do you suppose Joan is standing here this way?

M: [Response lost in the recording.]

E: All right. [Erickson now gives Joan a few directive touches and she responds by moving her hand and arm the exact amount indicated by his tactile cues.]

Now, the particular phenomenon that Joan is showing is this: Joan is perfectly willing to cooperate with me. She will put her hand down as far as I indicate; it stops moving when I indicate it by withdrawing my touch; it lowers as far as I indicate. But you take the person in the ordinary waking state—or you take the medical student who is deadset on faking a trance—and you ask him to show catalepsy: he shows it, surely enough, and you touch his hand gently and it goes [all the way to his lap on his side] over and over again even though you have told him. But after a while he will notice that he follows [your cues], and then you'll lift the other hand and that stays where you put it; and now he's really got a catalepsy there, because hypnotic phenomena are based one upon another.

R: A person faking tance will *interpret* Erickson's gentle touch as a cue to drop his hand all the way to his lap in one quick, smooth movement—as we usually do when we lower our hand in everyday life. The person experiencing genuine trance, however, will take Erickson's touch as a cue to move only as much as the touch indicates—no more and no less. The person in trance is responding in an exact and literal way to Erickson's touch cues. The faker presumes to interpret how he/she is supposed to move based on everyday rather than trance-type movements.

Recognizing Trance: Response Attentiveness; A General Posthypnotic Suggestion for Maximizing Potentials in Everyday Life

E: And if you'll look very carefully at Mary, you will notice a certain rigidity of her face, a certain loss of the blink reflex, a certain tremendous responsiveness and interest in what I am saying. . . . By the way, I'm talking to the audience, Mary. And you know that, do you not?

M: Yes.

E: Are you listening?

M: Uh-huh.

E: That's right, and it's good to listen. And I hope that you can understand me, and I hope that you can apply the particular learning that you acquire, physiologically and psychologically, to your own life in an exceedingly useful way.

R: Erickson now reviews the behavioral cues he is using to recognize that Mary has lapsed back into trance even though he asked her to rouse up. Recognizing that she is in a therapeutically responsive state, he then gives her a general and nonspecific posthypnotic suggestion to learn "physiologically and psychologically" what she can apply to her own life. Although he does this directly with such introductory phrases as "it's good to listen" and "I hope you can understand me," many professionals in the audience probably miss the fact that Erickson is actually giving a strong posthypnotic suggestion here.

Catalepsy Signaling the Persistence of Trance

Now I've lowered Joan's arm, but I didn't lower it in this sort of fashion [Erickson indicates a rapid, dismissive gesture to the audience with his other hand]. Therefore, it is still cataleptic. And you judge the persistence of a trance state by the continuance of certain hypnotic phenomena, and you can do it so gently and so easily and so unobtrusively. And Joan is standing there with her legs crossed, at ease, and her arm cataleptic.

Trance Awakening and Ratification: Hypnotic Amnesia to Overcome Learned Limitations

E: And now, Joan, I would like to have you take a deep breath and slowly rouse up. [Pause] That's right, hi! [Pause] How do you feel in front of this audience?

J: Fine.

E: Aren't you going to be shaky and tremulous?

J: No.

E: We'll let them be. [Laughter] Have you been in a trance?

J: I would say so.

E: You would say so. What happened while you were in a trance?

J: You were talking.

E: I was talking. What else?

J: I don't know.

E: Did you pay much attention to me, Joan?

J: Uh-huh.

E: Do you remember very well what I had to say?

J: Yeah.

E: Is it difficult to relate back?

J: No—I don't know. I was listening and at the time I remembered everything you said, but now I can't.

E: That's very nicely said, Joan, and that's what I hoped you would say. And I put my questions to you in such a way that it seemed to you that your answers might be just a little bit impolite. But they are truthful and they are informative. Yes, you were listening to me, and you heard and understood. But after you awakened there seemed to be some kind of a psychological distance. Isn't that right?

J: Uh-huh.

R: This was nicely said, indeed! There are two very important items to note in Joan's remarks here: (1) "I was listening and at the time I remembered everything you said" indicates that she was receiving what Erickson was saying while she was in trance; yet (2) she continues with "but now I can't." That is, she now has a hypnotic amnesia for what she knows she heard during trance. She has received the hypnotic suggestions; they are now lodged within her on an unconscious level but are no longer available to her conscious mind.

In a nutshell, this is the reason for the effectiveness of hypnotic suggestion. Patients have problems because of learned limitations; they have developed conscious mindsets that inhibit their conscious problem-solving efforts. By lodging suggestions on an unconscious level the unconscious has an opportunity to solve the problem unhindered by the conscious mind's limitations. Hypnotic amnesia seals the hypnotic suggestion within the womb of unconscious creativity.

The astute listener and reader will recognize how Erickson's questions actually facilitate the amnesia: "Do you remember *very well* what I had to say?", said in a subtle tone of doubt, certainly is an indirect suggestion not to remember; and "is it *difficult* to relate back?" also implies it will be difficult. So while most patients would experience hypnotic amnesia, thus ratifying their own trance experiences when it is brought to their attention, Erickson would typically reinforce the amnesia with indirect questions, the intent of which was usually not recognized by the subject—or in this case, not even by most of the professional audience.

Trance Deepening Via Questions: Behavioral Characteristics of Trance; The Narrowing and Focusing of Attention

E: And would you like to look at Mary right now? Now watch Mary's face, Joan. That's right, Mary. And how do you know when you are going into a trance, Mary? That's right, now can you verbalize it?

M: I listen to what you say. I take a deep breath—you suggested it.

E: You take a deep breath, and what else do you do?

M: I close my eyes. . . .

E: You close your eyes.

M: Relax.

E: But now as I talk and as you look at me and listen to what I say you're beginning to realize that you're going into a trance *without* taking a deep breath [voice softens], without closing your eyes. And perhaps you can tell us what you are doing. I don't know if you can, but I'm going to talk to the audience. And as you listen to me you can understand, and later you can tell me whether or not I'm right.

As she stands there listening to me with her eyes open and

without breathing deeply, there is a certain placidity of her face, there is a certain immobility of her face; there is that preliminary moving of her eyes around to take in the room, and then the slow, narrowing of the field of vision on me. And along with that slow narrowing of the field of vision on me there is a loss of responsiveness to the audience, a loss of responsiveness to all the rest of the room, and a slow forgetting of her hand and of her feet and of her shoulders.

R: When we left Mary a few sections back she was in a light trance receiving Erickson's posthypnotic suggestion for useful physiological and psychological learnings. Erickson now deepens that light trance with a classic question that indirectly facilitates trance induction and deepening: "And how do you know when you are going into a trance, Mary?" She can only answer this question by allowing sense memories of previous trances to be reactivated. As they are reactivated, of course, her trance deepens. Erickson then reviews for the audience the kind of observations that can be made to recognize trance behavior and the narrowing and focusing of attention.

Time and Trance Awakening: Muscle Tonus and Body Reorientation: Narrowed Attention as Not Sleep

E: Now close your eyes and take a deep breath, and rouse up and remember what I said.

And she's doing some of this so awfully nicely and so remarkably—something that you ought to study in the laboratory. And how much time is requisite for the individual to rouse from a trance? Now Mary has got her own sense of time. You should recognize that she has her sense of time in relationship to awakening from a trance. And if you watch very closely you'll see bit by bit the alteration in the muscle tonus; and at the right time I'll try to take advantage of it if I'm not facing the audience. But if a person takes a certain length of time in rousing more and more then you ought to recognize that certain people are going to take a certain amount of time in developing a trance.

E: Still more, Mary, and rousing more. That's right.

Now there is a slight head movement, there is a slight tendency to reorient the back of her head as it presses against the wall. And she is reorienting, I think, to her shoulders.

E: . . . . And slowly, gradually, open your eyes, rousing completely. That's right. That's right. Now, how accurately did I describe your behavior, Mary?

M: I think it's quite accurate, because I am paying attention to you.

E: You think it's quite accurate—

M: Yes, and I'm oblivious to my surroundings—

E: You're oblivious to your surroundings, and did you become aware of the back of your head against the wall?

M: Yes, yes.

E: Why?

M: Why? Well, you brought it to my attention, but with this hairdo, I feel even the slightest movement. [Laughter]

E: But, tell me—

M: I wasn't aware of it until you mentioned it, and then I realized—

E: All right, now which did you become aware of first,

your head or your shoulders against the wall?

M: My hair.

E: Your hair.

M: And then my shoulders.

E: And then your shoulders.

M: And then my face.

E: And then your face. That is, you more or less reassembled yourself.

M: Yes.

E: And which foot did you become acquainted with first?

M: I guess it was my right foot.

E: You guess it was your right foot, because you're not fully in contact with either, yet. Is that right?

M: I—I don't know. I haven't given it much thought.

E: You haven't given it much thought. Well, give it some thought.

M: [Pause] Yes, I have feet! [Much laughter]

E: Yes, that's right—you've got feet, now—two! [More laughter] Now, how did you learn to go into a trance?

M: Well, it's difficult because in a trance I expected to sleep. But I'm not asleep, I know what you're saying, and I feel myself relaxing—

E: But you're oblivious to the audience—

M: Because I'm paying attention to what you're saying.

E: In other words, you've narrowed your attention down.

R: The time required for trance induction and re-awakening, together with many of the behavioral characteristics of the latter process, are well illustrated in this section. Erickson felt it was imperative for student hypnotherapists to heighten their interpersonal sensitivity by making these observations of the idiosyncracies of patients and hypnotic subjects as they entered and awakened from trance. A grasp of these personal characteristics could greatly facilitate an understanding of patients' behavioral psychodynamics and thus facilitate future trance work.

Even in a nonhypnotic therapeutic interview, or in the casual affairs of daily life, the therapist will learn to observe the minimal behavioral signs of a person entering the common everyday trance (see *Experiencing Hypnosis)*. It is during such periods that most of us receive much of our unconscious conditioning as we receive the world and respond to it in a semiautomatic manner. We frequently have little amnesias for these light trance periods throughout the day (corresponding to the 90–120 minute ultradian cycle), and thus cannot understand later just how we could have done such-and-such or said such-and-such. This factor is emerging as especially important in the understanding of interpersonal relationships. Parents and children, teachers and students, men and women, all might find their interactions greatly enhanced by a careful regard for one another during these periods of blunted external awareness and heightened sensitivity to the inner world. When we learn to use the common everyday trance for the proper purposes, mutual understanding and support can only result.

Entering Trance without Awareness of It: Focusing Attention for Trance: Posthypnotic Suggestion Facilitating Human Potentials

E: Tell me, Joan, are you awake or in a trance?

J: Well, I think I'm awake—I feel awake.

E: You think you're awake, you feel as if you're awake. Tell me, do you think that Mary is awake?

J: Yes.

E: Why do you think she is awake?

J: Well, she just looks like she's awake.

E: Ohh. Now, you look at her and you tell me when Mary goes to sleep, will you? [Laughter] Now you watch Mary and you tell me when she is going asleep—because she is going to oblige you. [Pause] As soon as you feel reasonably confident, let me know. [Pause] You can do it, Joan, by winking with your right eye. You can let me know by slowly nodding your head up and down. Now keep watching her until you recognize that she is asleep.

Now here I've given Joan a very difficult task. Yet Joan has been in a trance, and sooner or later Joan will be able to appreciate when Mary goes into a trance. She may recognize it. And I've deliberately done something—I'll tell you about it later. [Long pause]

E: And is Mary in a trance, Joan?

J: I don't think completely.

E: You don't think completely. And you—

J: Am I in a trance?

E: Yes—[Pause] —are you in a trance?

J: I don't know.

E: You don't know.

Now what I did was to set up a situation in which Joan was forced to use learnings recently acquired at an unconscious level. What would she do? *She would try to re-establish the situation in which she had acquired those new learnings; therefore, she would tend to go into a trance without her awareness.* She has no objection, no unwillingness; she is perfectly agreeable to this situation, and so is Mary. And who is the important person in this situation? To Mary, it is Mary; to Joan, it is Joan. And Joan can look at Mary, but Joan is going to experience her own feelings, her own understandings; and Mary is going to experience *her* feelings, and be concerned about that. And both of them are going to have rapport with me and be responsive.

Now, how important is this type of technique? Do you really need a long, drawn-out, prolonged technique of induction? A medical student of mine is present in the audience who can remember when I put in a lot of time in prolonged techniques. But as I've become more experienced and more curious about the functioning of the mind, I've realized that not very much technique is necessary if you are willing to use your patient's attention. You need to focus it on some simple little thing and hold it there—like the single-mindedness of that little two-year-old who looked at the toy and wondered, "Just how can I get Mother to buy that for me?"—that utterly simple, single-mindednesss. And *you have a rather simple single-mindedness of purpose in trying to work toward your patients' welfare, knowing that you're not the final judge, knowing that you're not completely aware of the potentialities of the patients, but knowing that your patients ought to make every possible effort to achieve certain goals, and to be content with whatever achievement is within the limits of their possibilities.*

E: And that's right, isn't it Mary, that's right. And was I talking to the audience, Joan?

J: Yes.

E: That's right. And did you forget about the presence of the audience, Mary?

M: Yes.

E: Yes. It's very easy, isn't it?

M: Yes, it is.

E: And I would like to have you become interested in all of the things that you as a person can do in the utilization of your own physiological learnings, your own psychological learnings. I'd like to have you respect yourself as a human being with certain competencies and certain inadequacies such as we all possess; yours that make up your personality, that give you your individuality. And the same to you, Joan. I'd like to have both of you close your eyes. Mary, close your eyes and take a deep breath. Close your eyes, Joan, and take a deep breath. And feel very comfortable. And now take a deep breath and wake up wide awake and rested and refreshed. [Pause] Hi!

R: In this section Erickson illustrates the psychodynamics of entering an altered state without awareness of it. This is not only important as a technique of trance induction for therapeutic purposes, it is also a profound psychodynamic in everyday life that we are just beginning to become acquainted with.

Appropriate attitudes and expectations for the hypnotherapist are carefully summarized in the italicized section where we are cautioned to recognize our limitation in understanding the patient's potentials even while facilitating whatever possibilities are present. The unique individuality and inadequacies of each patient must be recognized. Not everyone can achieve the same level of hypnotic skills, but we each have a unique repertoire of potentialities that we need to discover by the continuing exploration of our nature. It is wise "to be content with whatever achievement is within the limits of their possibilities," because in the final analysis the patient and therapist's mutual wish for development via hypnosis faces the mutual limitations of their conscious understandings and points of view. The unconscious is still the vaster reservoir of wisdom in comparison with the conscious mind, and if the unconscious places restrictions on hypnotic achievement, then we must respect it even while continually probing to better understand why.

PART II

THERAPEUTIC USES OF
ALTERED ORIENTATION IN HYPNOSIS*

Since this is a sophisticated group it might be well to take up this matter of what hypnosis really is, of what you are really doing with your patients. Hypnosis occurs within the patient. The patient is only making responses to whatever stimulation you are offering. . . . You can tell a patient to stay awake, to stay wider awake, to stay very wide awake, and have him go into a profound trance. You can tell him to go to sleep, go very deeply asleep, and have him go into the same kind of profound trance. In other words, the hypnotic trance is something that occurs within the patient. It is a process of behavior in which patients alter their relationship to externalities; they alter their relationships to you and to whatever else is going on.

The patient who is sitting in a dental chair alters his relationship to external reality—to the window, the chair, and the furniture. All those items become tremendously unimportant. There is only one important thing for this patient in the dental chair, and that is the mouth. The patient gives attention to his mouth and to what the dentist is doing in his mouth. But the patient is giving that attention in a limited way. The patient does not feel [things irrelevant to the immediate situation], but he may experience a dry mouth very intensively.

The patient makes certain responses of a limited nature, or he may learn to alter habit patterns; but in all events he tempo-

*Workshop held in Los Angeles, California, May 2, 1962.

rarily forgets the things that govern everyday contacts. For example, all of you here now are fully conscious; none of you is in a trance state, and everyone of you is aware of the fact that I am sitting here at this table. You are aware of the fact, more or less continuously, that Dr. Steingart is here, that there is a loudspeaker over there, that there are lights in the ceiling, that the tablecloth is yellow. You don't need any of these generalized reality orientations in order to listen to me, or to follow your own trains of thought. Nevertheless, you have all been trained and conditioned biologically to check out your surroundings continuously—to look about you and discover where you are, what you are doing, who else is present—to reaffirm the fact that you are attending a lecture. That is important in our everyday working lives.

In hypnosis the patient has a totally different type of reality orientation. The patient can take an overall, comprehensive view of the situation and recognize it and understand it as much as is necessary. And having oriented in that one, comprehensive look to the surrounding reality, he can forget about it entirely until some major alteration of the surrounding reality comes in. The hypnotic subject recognizes nothing except major alterations.

Hypnotic and Reality Orientation in Obstetrics

It is therefore important that attention be given to that which the patient considers pertinent. It isn't important to an obstetrical patient how many nurses are in the room, how many doctors are in the room; it isn't important whether a surgical tray has been dropped. Nothing is important to the patient except the obstetrical situation and the patient's understanding of it.

Now this orientation of the hypnotic subject is a most important matter if you are going to use hypnosis successfully. What is the orientation of the pregnant woman on the delivery table? Well, all she really needs to know is that she is going to have a baby; and that in some way her pelvis is involved. But what if the obstetrical patient thinks that birth occurs *from the waist down?* If birth occurs *from the waist down,* that means her legs down to the soles of her feet are involved. If the obstetrician accidentally bumps against the knees, ankles, or feet, the patient will be disturbed because she includes her feet in that *below-the-waist* orientation.

I think you should recognize what kind of reality orientation the patient has. If you are an obstetrician, give your patient the understanding that her orientation should concern only her pelvic area; that the process of childbirth relates to the knowledge and the skill and the interest and the dexterity of the obstetrician; and that the patient can rely completely upon the birth canal and all that it includes.

Too often, the hypnotic situation breaks down because the patient's reality orientation is not comprehensive enough. The obstetrical patient should be told, directly or indirectly, that whatever happens in the delivery room is a legitimate part of the process of giving birth to a baby. When the patient understands that, the obstetrician is at liberty to do anything he finds advisable without distressing the patient.

Trance Induction by Utilizing Memories, Ideas and Concepts: Memories and Pain Relief

I stress the importance of understanding the patient's orientation to reality in order to facilitate hypnotic work. When you want to use hypnosis in dentistry, medicine, or psychological experimentation, you need to be aware of what it is your patient should include in the situation. A lot of the experimental work done in psychology laboratories has failed because the experimenter did not know what his subject was including in his orientation. Whether we are in the waking state or in the trance state, we tend to define reality according to our understandings.

As a dentist you need to define that reality situation for the patient so that the patient gives adequate attention to only those things that are important. How do you do that? Sometimes you do it by asking the patient to go down to the beach [in imagination] and enjoy a nice day while leaving his body behind in the office. Psychologically, you have oriented the patient as a functioning personality to the beach. That's safe enough—it's removed from the office; then everything that happens in the office is in relationship to the body being left behind. You have restricted and limited the patient's body orientation to the work that you are going to do.

Now this orientation on the part of the patient is spontaneous [and unconscious in the sense of not being premeditated]. Specifically, *you* need to discover the extent of the orientation and what its characteristics are. The more care you take in discovering this specific orientation to reality the more easily you will be able to induce a trance state; the more easily you will be able to get the patient to make trance responses; and [the more easily you will facilitate the] behavior that is essential to carry out your professional duties.

We learn from infancy to use reality in a certain way. But at the unconscious level we really are not concerned too much with concrete reality. When you look at a glass of water in the ordinary waking state you would like to *see* an actual glass of water; you like to see it held, you like to see its position, you like to see the extent of the water in the glass, and so forth. In the ordinary conscious state you are very, very dependent upon concrete reality. In the trance state, however, you can look at that glass of water right there [Erickson points to a vacant spot where there is no real glass of water], substituting for the actual glass a visual memory or a concept of what a glass of water is. [You make this substitution of the memory for the real] just as you use memories and concepts in dreams.

As soon as you recognize the tendency of the unconscious to rely upon memories, ideas, and concepts in place of concrete reality then it is much easier for you to ask your hypnotic subject to hallucinate. You're asking your patient to substitute for that state of pain the memory of a very pleasant feeling because in the unconscious there *is* a memory of a very pleasant feeling. All you want to do is take your patient's attention away from the concrete reality of the state of pain and direct it to that very real and very genuine concept or learning or memory or experience of comfort that exists within the unconscious mind.

You see, the patient himself has to do all the work. You can only offer a starting stimulus. At the races the starter fires the pistol, but it is the runner who wins the race. The firing of the pistol only announces the *beginning* of the race; it doesn't enter into the process of *running* the race. So it is with hypnosis. What the hypnotist says is like the firing of the pistol. The patient then has to do all of the "running" himself, and he can only do that in accordance with his own understandings.

How does the individual develop a trance state? Too many operators want a patient to become relaxed. It is a perfectly good way, but it also might be a perfectly wrong way for some particular patient. I can think of the patient suffering from extreme pain. You tell him to relax, but he is suffering from extreme pain and everything about him suggests extreme tension, anxiety, and attentiveness to pain. And you tell him to relax! That's simply talking nonsense because you are not paying attention to what hypnosis should mean to the patient. The proper approach to the patient suffering from extreme pain is *not* to suggest that he should be comfortable or relaxed. I tell the patient that he really *is* suffering from pain; that it really *does* hurt; and that he can notice that pain pretty thoroughly.

If it's a pain in the arm I am perfectly willing to point out to the patient that his arm really does hurt; and as surely as I do that I have narrowed his attention down to his arm. That's where I want his attention. I want that patient in pain to forget about this room, forget about those lamps, forget about this table ornament, forget about the tablecloth. I want the patient to become aware of his arm, and as soon as he becomes aware of that painful arm exclusively, then that patient is in a position to remember that this pain now is really different from that former feeling of comfort in his arm. So now I have the patient thinking about comfort as well as pain. . . . He knows that I am not discrediting his pain; that I am not doubting it. I'm emphasizing his pain and he knows that I respect it. Therefore, when I tell him he has a past history of comfort and ease where he has that pain he is going to respect my statement and he is going to know it is true. Then he is going to establish that abstract mental reality of comfort and ease in his arm within himself.

As soon as you introduce the memories of comfort and ease

into a pain situation the pain begins to diminish because you have only so much attention to give. You can give all of your attention to the pain, or you can give most of it to the pain and a little of it to the memories of comfort and ease. Then you can give progressively more and more attention to the ease and comfort, and less and less attention to the pain. [But to immediately suggest relaxation when the patient is in extreme pain is to invite failure.]

Utilizing the Patient's Behavior: The Hyperactive Child

You need to think about the manner of feeling, thinking, and emotion the patient has in relationship to the reality of his body and his body experiences at the moment. This morning I was asked a question about the child who comes into the office and races back and forth and is awfully uncooperative. My answer was rather simple. The first thing I would recognize about that child is that his reality is one of racing back and forth; it is one of not cooperating with me. You see that the child is carrying out some motor activity. I think the child had better keep right on carrying out that motor activity because that child needs to work with me. How should the child work with me?

I tell him, "You are running to this door; you are running up here and you are running toward that door; to this door over here, and back again to that door."

The first thing the child knows he is actually *waiting* for me to tell him which way to run. If the child starts fighting with me [Erickson gestures to demonstrate a pushing motion] I may tell him how now he is pushing with his right hand, then with his left hand. The first thing you know, the child is waiting for me to say, "Push me off with your right hand; now push me off with the left hand"! In other words, the therapist learns to utilize patients' personal orientations to their situations. You should bear in mind that it's the patients' own mental processes that allow them to do so.

What Is Hypnotic Behavior?
Three Temper Tantrums of Miss O:
Spontaneous Hypnosis and Age Regression*

Hypnosis is not something that comes about by a traditional ritualistic method. People can develop hypnosis spontaneously if you give them half a chance. This matter of spontaneous hypnosis occurred in the first seminar on hypnosis held in the United States, conducted by Clark L. Hull at the University of Wisconsin, in September, 1923. Dr. Hull, who later became President of the American Psychological Association, had told me that if I would spend the summer doing experimental work in hypnosis and report on it, then he would conduct a seminar. I agreed.

One of the members of that seminar was Miss O. Miss O and I soon got acquainted and [she told me a bit about her family background]. She had been an only child and was rather badly spoiled. She had had one particular idiosyncrasy: she *had* to have her own way. Her usual manner of getting her own way had been to do the following: She would enter her house, stomp her feet upon meeting her mother, make her demands, throw a temper tantrum, race upstairs into her bedroom, throw herself on her bed, and burst into sobs. Long experience and practice had taught Miss O that she could really govern her parents in this particular fashion.

I asked Miss O if she would mind the seminar group knowing about this, and she had no hesitation telling them.

Now that seminar on hypnosis was really a seminar on human behavior. The questions we raised were: What constitutes hypnotic behavior?; What are the processes involved?; How does hypnosis come about?; What happens when you do this thing or that thing? [To find answers to these questions I proposed the following experiment:]

I pointed out that our seminar room was just at the head of

Editors' Note: See "Further Experimental Investigations of Hypnosis: Hypnotic and Nonhypnotic Realities," *Collected Papers,* Vol. 1, pp. 18-82.

the stairway, and that we had a nice table. I proposed to Miss O that she go downstairs to the first floor, go over to the side door, open it, step outside, close the door, and then reopen it. Next she was to come inside, stomp her feet, race up the stairway, enter the seminar room, slam the door behind her, and come over to the seminar table where her chair was. What we really wanted to know in all of this was what would happen when Miss O reenacted her childhood pattern of temper tantrums.

Now Miss O was intelligent and scientific-minded, and very willingly agreed to the experiment. She went downstairs, stepped outside the side door, thought the matter over, smiled to herself, came inside, looked up and down the hallway to see if the other students were present, stomped her feet, came racing up the stairs, slammed the seminar door shut, flung herself into her chair, lowered her head in her arms, and burst into violent sobbing.

After some minutes of sobbing (during which time the group remained too amazed to do anything), Miss O straightened up and curiously turned to berate me for the outrageous suggestion that I had given her. Then she really launched into a tirade denouncing the entire seminar group. It was the most beautiful display of uncontrolled temper you ever saw.

She finally cooled down and said, "I got angry." She was as much surprised as the rest of us.

We discussed it again and then one of us raised the question to Miss O, "Where did you start getting angry?"

Miss O said simply, "I don't remember."

Next we suggested to her, "Why don't you do it all over again and see at what point you get angry?"

So Miss O went downstairs and repeated the entire episode. The second time she burst into the room she really slammed that door, flung herself down, repeated the whole scene, cussed me out, cussed the group out, and then in the excitement said, "I got angry again!"

We asked her, "Where did you start getting angry?"

Miss O said, "I was wondering about that as I raced up the stairs. I started to get angry when I was about halfway up the

stairs, but I don't remember anything after that halfway point."
Then we suggested, "Suppose you go downstairs and do it
all over again."

To our surprise, Miss O said, "Well, I don't think I would
have to go all the way downstairs."

She got up, went over and opened the seminar door, saying,
"Well, I don't have to go downstairs."

She then slammed the door, threw herself back into her seat,
and proceeded into her third tantrum.

We speak about regression. We speak about the re-establish-
ment of previous patterns of reaction. Here was an ordinary
postgraduate seminar in which an earnest person was asked
whether or not she would be able to re-establish a previous pattern of behavior. . . . We did a little experimenting with various
other people, asking them if they could do that sort of thing,
and we found that a number of them could reenact a scene
from their past experiences in which they would actually regress, having no real control over their behavior.

Now, what is the relationship of all this to hypnosis?: You
use hypnosis exactly in that same sort of way.

Altered States in Hypnosis and Introspection: The Introspection Experiment*

I conducted another experiment to find out what manner of
behavior enters into this question of hypnosis. I set up an experiment using engineering students, agriculture students, and
English students. Now I was just a pre-med student at the time,
and I didn't have prestige of any sort, and so I set up an experiment which I explained as an investigation of the processes by
which one does some thinking. I explained to my subjects that
what I wanted them to do was to volunteer for an experiment
in the psychology department to see if they could figure out the
processes by which they did a certain amount of thinking. I got

*See "Initial Experiments Investigating the Nature of Hypnosis," *Col-
lected Papers,* Vol. I, pp. 3–17.

a few dozen students to volunteer, all sorts of students, male and female.

Now, the experiment went as follows. [First, I would explain matters to the subject:]

"We have this chair. It is a nice, comfortable chair. I want you to sit in it with your hands on your lap and be comfortable. I want you mentally to think through the processes that would be involved if you were to take your right hand or your left hand, reach over to that imaginary basket of fruit on that imaginary table, pick up an imaginary apple, and put it on the table in front of you.

"In thinking all that through, you will first have to start with thinking: 'My hand is in my lap. To pick up an apple over there I'll have to lift my hand, and that means I'll have to bend my elbow—which means I'll have to lift my elbow—which means I'll have to lift my forearm—which means I'll have to lower my hand—which means I'll have to feel the apple with my fingertips.' You, yourself, can think through that process."

The subjects were to sense everything. They were to go through thoroughly the mental processes of seeing their arms reaching over there, feeling different in the shoulders, seeing their hands reach over to the table in front of them, seeing the apple.

"What are all the thoughts that go through your mind? How much attention would you pay to the smell of the apple? How much would you notice how very red it is?"

A number of the subjects would try to carry out the visualization but after a few minutes of effort would declare the task an impossible one and state emphatically that they were disgusted. Others tried very hard, but kept asking for encouragement and further instructions. I would tell these subjects that it was *their* thinking that was important, not mine.

Certain other subjects would really start to think. You could see that they were tremendously interested in what they were doing until suddenly, in a shocked reaction, they would say something like: "I'm beginning to feel funny all over. I feel awfully funny. I'm getting out of here." And they would!

There were still other subjects who didn't mind feeling "funny all over," and they would go through the mental process of picking up the apple and putting it on the table. Now everyone of these subjects who went through the mental process, step by step, of picking up the apple and putting it on the table felt "funny." *That funny feeling was the process of going through a trance stage; it was the loss of orientation to external reality and the establishment of an abstract conceptual reality....* Yet the words *hypnosis* and *suggestion* were never spoken. All I was interested in purportedly was the process of thinking and understanding that one goes through in order to imagine picking up an apple and putting it on a table in front of one.

I later looked up all the students who had gotten that shock reaction, had complained of feeling "funny," and had said, "I'm getting out of here!" I now told them that I was interested in hypnosis and requested that they participate in a hypnotic induction. They all reported that the "funny" feeling they had experienced in the introspection experiment was just like the hypnotic feeling in trance. In other words, the subjects recognized the different orientation [that exists in hypnosis and many hypnotically absorbing tasks].

I think this matter of orientation to reality is going to play a significant role in space methods. I think the astronauts in space will find the loss of gravity to be an initially interesting, charming, and pleasing experience. But what are they going to do when they have lost that feeling of riding by the seat of their pants in normal gravity? They will lose a lot of orientation; they won't know how to orient their bodies. That's exactly what you do with hypnotic subjects. You take away their reality orientation just as I did with subjects down at the Aeronautical Space Medical Laboratories. Those subjects felt very, very distressed within about twenty or thirty minutes of sitting in chairs, not knowing whether they were sitting in chairs on the floor, the ceiling, or the wall. They had lost their sense of spatial orientation.

Light and Deep Trance Simultaneously: "Calloused" Pain Nerves

It is your patient's reality orientation that allows you to deal with his anxieties and muscular patterns. It certainly aids you to understand what kind of a reality orientation your patient brings into the office for you to deal with. *As surely as you recognize what the patient's orientation is you can set up the therapeutic situation.* I will give you an example.

Not very long ago, a California physician had been treating a woman for chronic pain. He had consulted various other physicians before calling me in on the case. The woman gave every evidence of pain, but all the medical and neurological examinations indicated no organic basis for it. Still, there was no question about the woman's total behavior: she was suffering serious, chronic pain.

What are you going to do with this type of patient? Hypnosis had been used without success. The woman had little or no faith in hypnosis *as she understood it.* Before she came into my office she wanted to know if I was going to use hypnosis on her. I recognized the question immediately as an antagonistic, resistful one. My reply was: "We'll use anything that is necessary. We won't use anything that isn't necessary."

In other words, by emphasizing the fact that I wouldn't use anything that wasn't really necessary I made her recognize that whatever I did would be pertinent.

How deep a trance can you induce in someone who would be intensely alert, aware, and observant, looking in all directions to see what I would be doing next. My feeling was to use so light a degree of trance that the patient would not detect that I was using hypnosis at all. Therefore, what I did was to get her to intensify the pain in her hips along the course of her sciatic nerve; I asked her to pay full attention to it; I asked her to observe that pain studiously. As I explained it to her:

"You have had the pain for so long and you hate it so much that you'd rather not know its various attributes. But I want to know every one of the attributes of that pain. And I would like to have that pain become utterly excruciating, terribly intense, so that you will really know whether it's a burning pain, a cutting pain, a lancinating pain." And I ran off a whole series of adjectives.

Next, I summarized by saying, "But I would like to have you describe that pain in your own words and not try to put it in medical terms."

I got the woman so interested in sitting quietly and mentally studying the pain in her right hip and along the course of her right sciatic nerve that I think my secretary could have come in and played the drums and the patient wouldn't have noticed. She was really absorbed, yet she would notice immediately if I rustled a piece of paper; she knew if I looked at my watch; she knew if I wrote something in the case record. But she was unobservant for everything else in the office.

As far as I was concerned, as far as the therapeutic situation was concerned, this woman was in an utterly light trance. But in relation to alien reality, to *irrelevant* reality, she was in a very profound trance because she was so completely inattentive to it. I stress this distinction because *it is very important for you to recognize that your patient can be in a very light trance and in a very deep trance at the same time*—in a light trance in relation to one part of reality, and in a deep trance in relation to another part of reality. It is your obligation to be aware of these differences so that when you want to deal with fear or anxiety or pain or distress you can partition off that reality in which your patient is going to learn; that pattern of behavior that the patient comes to learn from you.

This patient really studied her pain; she really described it to me fully. I then told her I would like to explain the origin, genesis, development, and reason for the persistence of the pain; that if she were willing to listen to me, I would try to explain slowly and carefully and gently and in nonmedical terms so that she could understand.

Well, I wouldn't want a medical man to read the things I said to that woman! I pointed out to her some awfully unscientific things. But she did not come to get an education in neurology, in psychology, or in any other science. She came for relief of pain. I pointed out to her that just as you can have all kinds of habits—you can have mouth habits such as tongue thrusting or teeth grinding, you can have speech habits such as stuttering or stammering, and you can have eating habits and olfactory habits and gustatory habits—*so also can you have pain habits.* You can take various stimuli and habitually translate them into pain responses. [And you can also learn to do the reverse.]

Actually, this is true. Consider the first time you ate Mexican food: you blew the flames out, you drank cold water—anything to put out the fire in your mouth. Yet any little Mexican child can tell you how completely delightful the food is. Once you had learned to translate the stimulation of the pepper into a pleasant sensation you, too, found Mexican food to be utterly delightful.

I put that sort of understanding into my patient's chronic pain, and for the first time she began to realize that she had some new learnings to acquire about pain. I pointed out to her that if I went into my garden and hoed for an hour, I would have blisters on both my hands. If I then waited a couple of weeks until my hands healed, went back out to hoe for another hour or two, I would again end up with blisters on my hands. But if I went out today and hoed for thirty seconds, went out tomorrow and hoed for forty seconds, and in such a manner gradually increased the work by a minute at a time, soon I would be able to hoe all day long without getting blisters because I would have developed a callous formation.

I pointed out that the first time you eat Mexican food without any callous formation on your tongue or on your lips, you really feel it. But after you get the proper callous formation, you can really eat that Mexican food. You have a callous formation that cuts out all the pain while your taste buds remain sensitive to the delightful flavor of Mexican food.

In such a way I raised this matter of callous formation of pain nerves for my patient. I know that callous formation is a rather unscientific analogy, but this woman wanted some understanding that would help her. I pointed out to her that she really ought to be willing to spend the same length of time developing nerve callouses down her hip as I would be willing to spend putting callouses on the palms of my hands in order to hoe, or on my tongue in order to eat that highly spiced Mexican food. She sat there listening to me, attentive to the fact that every time I picked up a pencil she was able to perceive it; every time I looked at the clock, every time I shifted my gaze, she was fully aware of it. But she was wonderfully unaware of the rest of the office. She listened and she absorbed those ideas I presented.

I spent two hours with her and then sent her home. Her family physician spoke with me last Sunday and wanted to know what on earth I had done. Apparently, my patient had not waited a month to develop those calluses. She arrived home from Phoenix free of pain and very proud of the fact that somehow she was managing to translate the experience of pain into a feeling of comfort. Now, I would have failed with this particular patient if I had attempted to diminish her pain by directly inducing an anesthesia or an analgesia. She had an orientation that pain fit into her reality. [I helped her utilize that reality in a manner that allowed her to experience comfort as well.]

Accepting the Patient's Reality: A Cardiac Neurosis

I'm thinking of a man I saw not long ago. His cardiologist had phoned me and said: "I am sending you a patient. The electrocardiogram is normal. The man has a cardiac neurosis. You had better handle him. I can't."

When the man came into my office he was sobbing and yelling, "I'm scared! I'm scared! Something is going to happen— I'm afraid I'm going to die of heart failure!"

He was frightened, he was trembling all over. At home he had been having hysterical seizures similar in intensity to epileptic seizures.

As soon as he had come into my office I told him, "When you go to sit down, I would like to have you sit crosswise in the chair; that way, when you faint or have a seizure you can fall in that direction, because I don't want your head bumping against the bookcases over here."

Now, that was thoughtfulness on my part. The patient was extremely fearful. Why should I tell him that he wouldn't faint? Why should I tell him that he wouldn't have a seizure? Why

113

shouldn't I take it for granted that he *would* do all those things? Only then will the patient know that I truly understand his reality. The cardiologist had tried to tell this patient things that were contrary to the patient's experiences. Therefore, the cardiologist got nowhere.

The patient sat crosswise in the chair as I had asked. I pointed out to him that an hour was a rather short period of time, and that I noticed that his breathing was reasonably comfortable. So he began to notice his breathing, and it was reasonably comfortable.

Then I pointed out, "Along with easy breathing, of course, you know you have an *easier* heart rate."

I didn't say *easy* heart rate. I said *easier*. He could accept that, and he began looking at the reality of his own heartbeat. Well, it didn't take very long to get that patient to decide I really understood his case.

Too many therapists try to reassure patients; they try to deprive their patients of the reality of their symptoms [rather than accepting and working with that reality].

If a patient walked into your office and said, "My arm is broken," and you could see angulation in the forearm, can you imagine responding: "Now, sit down; maybe you are mistaken; maybe you haven't a broken arm; you haven't really got a broken arm!" The patient would walk out of your office and get a physician who could see and admit an angulation of that forearm.

Yet doctors will tell patients, "Now you don't need to worry; you don't need to be afraid; you really don't need to be anxious."

[What are you doing with that kind of approach?] You are denying and rejecting something that is as real to the patient as a broken arm is. You need to orient your thinking along these lines. As surely as you let the patient know that you have as much respect for his fear, his anxieties, and nervousness as you have for his broken arm or for his broken jaw, then that patient will recognize that you understand him. As soon as the patient recognizes that you understand his symptoms, that you understand what the condition is, that you are willing to deal with that condition *as it is,* then the patient can take his reality orientation and focus it down to where it should be.

A Hypnotic Approach with Children: The Traumatic Scratch

I am thinking of a little neighbor girl who rushed in to see me one day because I am a doctor. She had what she thought was a great big bad cut on her leg, just above the knee. She was crying, she was frightened, she wanted me to do something about it.

She pleaded, "You are a doctor, you've got to do something about my cut—it hurts—it's awful!"

I told here, "It hurts awful right there," and she agreed. It did hurt awful right *there* and I pointed to that tiny little scratch as I saw it. I continued:

"It hurts awful right *there.* It doesn't hurt right here, half an inch to one side. It doesn't hurt here, half an inch to the other side. Just right *there.* And it hurts from here to here," and I pointed to the full length of that one-inch-long scratch.

That little girl knew that I really understood her situation, so next I said, "Now we can go to work and stop the hurt."

I had won that girl's absolute confidence, for I had recognized that her cut hurt awfully. But it didn't hurt here, didn't hurt there. It hurt just right *there,* and all the way from here up to there. I had narrowed the girl's reality orientation down to that inch-long scratch, and so the two of us could go to work and take the hurt away. Since she was a child, only a few words of suggestion were necessary to remove the hurt. She didn't even want a Band-Aid, even though I offered her various colors of them to wear. The scratch wasn't bad enough; the fright was pretty bad, but the fright would go away.

Now, what kind of a trance did I have her in? I would say a very light one, but as far as her hurt was concerned it was really a very deep trance.

In the practice of dentistry you want your patient in a very deep trance orally but in a very light trance in other regards. In this matter of fear and anxiety you try to center the patient's attention on it by your acknowledgment of this symptomatology—of his fears and anxieties. You never try to discredit what the patient knows is a reality for him.

Hallucinations and Rapport: The Floating Nude Men

I can think of a patient some years ago who walked into my office—followed by half a dozen young, nude men who had tailed her, floating in midair, all over the city of Phoenix! When she mentioned this situation to me I recognized that she was as psychotic as it was possible to be. Before she got all the way into my office, she noticed that I had a big, steel, bear trap set in the middle of the floor. She walked around it, asking if I thought it sensible or reasonable to keep a bear trap set on the floor of my office. I told her I didn't really think it was reasonable, that I thought something should be done about it, and would she mind walking around it.

Next, the patient discovered that I kept half a dozen nude dancing girls in the corner of my office, and she began to worry that her young men would fraternize with those young girls of mine. I told her that I would see to it that my dancing girls did not fraternize with her young men.

Why should I dispute that patient's delusions and hallucinations? They were hers. I had better respect them in the same way I respect a broken leg or a broken jaw. Knowing that I respected her hallucinations and her delusions, that woman was able to develop a rapport with me; she was able to go into a trance: Eventually she was able to teach in a high school, to function as a successful counselor, and, years later, to function as a secretary to the president of a large corporation. [You really ought to accept and utilize the patient's reality.]

Approaches to Dental Problems: Division and Awareness for Habit Problems: Thumbsucking

Let's discuss this matter of treating harmful dental habits—neuromuscular habits such as gagging, thumb sucking, and bruxism. I'm thinking of a doctor's son I knew who was six years old at the time. The doctor had told his son of all the ills that would be his if he didn't stop sucking his thumb. The child's mother was a nurse and she told him of all the ills that would be his. [But the child continued to suck his thumb.] Finally, they brought the boy to me.

I began by asking the parents to exercise professional ethics by acknowledging that their son was my patient and that I didn't want either one of them interfering with my therapy in any way. Then, little Jimmy came in to see me. I told him right off:

"Your father and mother want you to stop sucking your thumb, and they told you that they were going to bring you to me to make you stop. I'd like you to understand one thing: your thumb is your thumb; your mouth is your mouth. If you want to suck your thumb, you go right ahead. Your Daddy can't boss me; your Mommy can't boss me; and I'm not going to boss you. *But if you want to, you can boss your thumb, and you can boss your mouth, and you can go ahead and suck your thumb as much as you like.*"

I'd better recognize that six-year-old boy's reality. He didn't expect me to say what I said to him. He expected me to interfere. Adult patients also expect you to interfere with their symptomatology, with their bad habits. I think it is awfully important for you to recognize the reality orientation of your patients.

Little Jimmy stood back rather astonished, and then he tested me by putting his thumb into his mouth. I pointed out to him that I thought it awfully unfair that he sucked only his left thumb; that his right thumb was just as nice a thumb and it was entitled to just as much sucking, and that I was astonished [that he wasn't sucking his right thumb as well]. Little Jimmy thought that he was at fault. Being a nice, bright boy, Jimmy should be willing to suck *both* thumbs. But, you see, what happens is that as surely as Jimmy sucks *both* thumbs he has cut down sucking his left thumb by about fifty per cent. He has reduced his habit. And what about that forefinger, and the other three fingers?: *When you start dividing, you start conquering.*

117

Then I pointed out to Jimmy that in a couple of months he was going to be seven years old. No longer a mere six. He would be joining the big kids when he turned seven years old.

"And you know, Jimmy, I don't know a single big kid that sucks his thumb, so you'd better do plenty of thumb sucking before you join the big kids. You'd really better get plenty of it."

I confronted Jimmy with the laborious task of really getting enough thumb sucking in before he joined the big kids. And he wanted to join the big kids; he didn't want to be a mere six-year-old. Every six-year-old wants to be a seven-year-old. The essential thing is to join with the child in appreciating his concept of his reality.

Gagging

In this matter of gagging, why not be perfectly honest with your patient by telling him, "You really do gag." I know it, and he knows it, and I'd better know that he knows it. Then I can ask the patient to really study that gag: Where does the gagging really start—in the abdomen, in the thorax, in the pharynx?; where do you really get that feeling first? You ask the patient to focus on his gagging.

I think I have given this illustration to you before, and yet it is worth repeating. *Whenever you start picking things apart, you destroy them. You destroy their value.* A pretty girl is very kissable. Look at that pretty girl and you see she has such a kissable face. But look closer and, of course, her eyes are a little too close together—her ears are a little bit too large—her nose is slightly long—her chin is pretty heavy—that lower lip is really too thick—her mouth is really too wide. Who wants to kiss her once you pick that face apart! You pick a pain apart, you pick gagging apart, you pick nausea apart, you pick fear apart, you pick anxiety apart—all in exactly the same sort of way.

Tongue Habits

Let's discuss this matter of swallowing. Ogden Nash wrote a very nice poem about the centipede. The centipede was walking

118

along perfectly happily one day, with all of his legs going in proper order, until along came so-and-so who asked the centipede which leg came after which. Now that poor centipede lies in a ditch wondering which comes after which.

You ask the patient with a lot of bad tongue habits if he would like to discover something about his tongue habits. Then you point out that he really has certain tongue habits. How many patients actually recognize what a tongue habit is—what a muscle habit is—what a speech habit is? Most patients don't recognize these matters at all.

You try to tell a person the right place to put the tongue in order to swallow properly. But your patient has had years of training, years of experience, in putting his tongue in a different place. He tries to put it in a different place, in the place you recommend, but he automatically puts his tongue in the usual place and gets a tongue thrust, or some other faulty movement. The patient needs to learn to recognize individual tongue movements and how to coordinate them. In other words, you really ought to help him pick apart that tongue movement.

How many different movements of the tongue are possible? Take a mirror and hold it in front of yourself: You can narrow your tongue, you can curve your tongue, you can widen your tongue; you can extend it, you can pull it back, you can curl up the tip of it. You can get the patient interested *not* in his tongue thrust, but in the habit and in the form and in the structure of the various tongue movements that are possible. You ask the patient to become aware that he can widen his tongue, he can narrow it, he can curl the tip, he can fold it over, and maybe he can even touch his nose with it. You teach him that he has a certain dexterity with his tongue.

Consider the situation of the child who says that he cannot stop putting his tongue tip against his upper teeth: He says that he tries and tries, but his tongue always gets up there and he simply can't stop it. Why shouldn't you agree? He knows he has had experience with his tongue; it is his mouth. But as surely as you start disputing him about what he does with it you are lost.

Now you ask him to focus his reality orientation on his mouth. He doesn't need to look out of the window, but he does need to look in his mouth and see if he can put that tongue of his against the molars. Can he really put it against the molars? Right side, left side? In other words, *you teach the child how to make purposeful tongue thrusts;* you teach him to thrust his tongue against the rear molars, against the premolars, the canines, the incisors, the uppers, the lowers. You teach him to tongue thrust against all the teeth he has, and to count his teeth in that way. You haven't taken away his privilege of thrusting his tongue against his incisors, but you have added to that tongue thrust a lot of other tongue thrusting so that *the pathological tongue thrust becomes a minor percent of a total muscle pattern.*

Traumas and Phobias

Consider the child who is afraid of dogs, awfully afraid of dogs, especially of that *great big brown dog.* She is really terrified of dogs and of their barking. Certainly you find out all about her feelings and you do not discredit any one of them. You center her attention down and down and down to that bite the *great big brown dog* gave her on her knee; to the bite he gave her on her face; to the fact that the dog wasn't barking when he bit her on the face; he wasn't barking when he bit her on the knee; that he was a *big* dog, not a little dog; that he was a *great big brown dog,* not a little willy black dog. And you are constantly emphasizing this girl's reality to the *great big brown dog* that bit her; to that one dog that bit her on the face and bit her on the knee. You take her all-inclusive, comprehensive, phobic reaction to dogs in general and you narrow it down [to the dog that actually bit her]. [You are taking an important step toward symptom relief] by asking that patient to clarify for you her experience of reality. As she tells you all about that *great big brown dog* she cuts her problem down to the point where she can tell you that your *big short-legged brown dog* is a nice dog, because he is not a *great big brown dog.* [You can gradually add more distinctions until the generalized phobia is reduced back to the original fright which is no longer a problem since no current reality can exactly match the past.]

Bruxism

Anyone who treats bruxism should check first with the dentist as to the cause of it. I expect that whenever you treat a patient for a condition you first carry out a thorough physical examination, no matter what the condition is, so that you are treating the patient for what is really the problem. Why should you believe what the patient says is the problem? The patient can come in and tell you that she has ulcers of the stomach when the reality is that she is pregnant. Then you had better know that the patient is pregnant. She is unexpectedly pregnant; she has been married for fifteen years and has been unable to get pregnant. Now she starts vomiting, she has a pain in her stomach, and she thinks she is developing ulcers. Now this was an actual case of mine, and as I listened to that woman I made my own diagnosis. I did not accept her diagnosis.

In bruxism you ought to know the facts from the dentist's point of view. If there is something pathological about the teeth that causes the bruxism, let the dentist correct it with dental tools. If it's a psychological matter, if it's a pattern of behavior, then you want to correct it with psychological tools.

The patient may tell you: "But I don't grind my teeth. I don't care what my wife says, I don't care what my sister says, I don't care what my brother says, *I don't grind my teeth."*

Being a dentist, you look in the mouth and you have your own suspicions about whether or not the teeth are being ground. How are you going to orient the patient? You ought to be willing to recognize that the patient who grinds his teeth at night is trying to deceive and deny. If he grinds his teeth he ought to have certain jaw responses and jaw memories, certain body memories and body understandings. Your own reality orientation should tell you that.

The patient says again, "But I don't grind my teeth! I don't care what my brother says or my mother says, or anyone says, *I just don't grind my teeth."*

You can wonder what kind of feeling the patient really has that made his mother or his brother or whoever make such an idiotic mistake as to think that he was grinding his teeth. What kind of feelings does he have in his jaw? Maybe they mistook peculiar kinds of jaw movement for teeth-grinding movements. What are the jaw movements that you can make? You get the patient interested in that particular question. To do this, do you need a somnambulistic trance, or do you need a light trance, or do you simply need the patient oriented to this question: What kinds of movements do you make with your jaw; how many different kinds of movements are *possible* with your jaw?

I can think of a woman who said that her eating pattern was perfectly in order. But her dentist told her that she had a bad bite. Then the woman got another dentist [who told her that her bite was fine]. I thought the first dentist was probably correct, but I initially accepted her point of view and pondered with her why the first dentist had made such a ridiculous assertion. She went on to tell me that the first dentist had said something about a bad bite causing her pain around the side of her head. The woman admitted that she did have temple pain, but she associated it with headaches, not with her eating. So I went into the question of how the jaw works while chewing. We really got involved in this matter of jaw movement while eating: how you eat differently when the steak is tough than when the steak is tender; how you use your jaw to crack walnuts open (if you are so unwise as to use your teeth for such a maneuver in the first place); and just exactly what sort of thinking you have as you slip that walnut into your mouth.

As I asked these questions I carefully watched to see if she were left- or right-sided in her chewing orientation. I asked the woman a goodly number of questions, and then I pointed out to her the spontaneous location of everything to the right side of her mouth.* I suggested that she go through the process of imagining herself setting a piece of very tough steak in her

Editors' Note: Erickson always watched patients very carefully whenever he asked them questions about their body behaviors. As the patients reflected on the question, they usually made minute body movements (in this case, chewing on the right side) that revealed how their bodies actually behaved in reality.

mouth and then eating it. Once she realized that she did do most of her chewing on the right side of her mouth, she decided that the first dentist *did* know what he was talking about, and that she really ought to go back to him.

Is this hypnosis, or is it simply the correction of the patient's orientation? In bruxism, as with many other symptoms, you ask patients to consider their habits and their various muscle movements.

Dancing Instructions:
Body Awareness and Muscle Sensations

A patient came to see me and said, "I can't possibly learn to dance—I've taken Arthur Murray lessons and I've got three left feet!"

I asked this man if he could take up just one foot at a time, and for convenience sake, let's take the left foot first.

"What feelings would you have if you were to lift your foot up and put it down one step ahead; and then if you were to move it slightly to one side, and then move it slightly back."

I got him tremendously interested in the feeling of that left foot. Then I asked him to stand up and describe the feelings to me again, but this time while demonstrating as well:

"Put your left foot forth, and describe the feeling to me; next, move the left foot to one side; now move it back again; now put it behind your right foot; now move it ahead again, all the while describing the feelings in that foot to me."

Well, the man has since learned to dance just finely, and he now has only two feet—one right and one left! It was a matter of asking him to study the reality of his own muscle sensations.

Subtle Negative Suggestion with Children

Let's return to this matter of bruxism. I think as soon as the child is old enough you really ought to take up with him the question of the feelings in his mouth, and the question of how the mouth works. Once you get the child interested in his own bruxism movement, sooner or later he will show it to you. You ask him really to memorize those feelings, and then you express the very pious hope that he *won't* awaken when he makes that bruxism movement during sleep. And you express this hope so nicely and so genuinely and so suggestively that you actually condition him to awaken by your subtle negative suggestion. You can also suggest that he will be able to *hear* the bruxism; that he will awaken when he hears it; and that he will immediately comfort himself with the realization that he has a good pattern of going back to sleep whenever he awakens. But how many times does a person want to awaken in the middle of the night just to prove to himself that he can hear his bruxism, and that he can go right back to sleep! You select out of the patient's reality that part of it that is useful in correcting his faulty habit.

Attitudes and Life Experiences of the Therapist as Determinants for Patient Responses

It is your attitude toward the patient that determines the results you achieve. Now, I don't know how many times I have demonstrated this point in seminars. I do know that I've demonstrated it experimentally with my medical students time and time again.* In the experiment, I told Group A of my medical students that a certain subject was an excellent hypnotic subject, except that *she could not develop anesthesia or analgesia;* I told Group B of my medical students that she was an excellent hypnotic subject and that she could develop every phenomenon *except visual hallucination;* and I told the third group that she could develop everything *except auditory hallucination.* In actual fact, *the young lady was able to develop all the hypnotic phenomena.*

As it turned out, each group achieved different results with this subject. When I asked Group A for a report, they said that they had gotten every possible phenomenon from her *except anesthesia and analgesia.* The second group, listening, had said, "What on earth is the matter with you! She develops anesthesia

*See *Collected Papers,* Vol. II.

124

and analgesia, but *she doesn't develop visual hallucination.*"
Then the third group intervened, "She develops visual hallucination and anesthesia, but *she doesn't develop auditory hallucination!*"

After all this I brought the subject in and asked her to tell the students what my instructions to her had been. I had said something like the following: "Various groups of medical students are going to work with you. I want you to do *whatever they really mean.*" My subject then explained how "this young medical student told me to develop glove anesthesia, but he didn't mean it. He didn't really expect me to do it. That medical student asked me to develop visual hallucination, but he didn't really mean it. He didn't believe I could. *So I didn't.*"

Several years ago my daughter was at a seminar, and she very carefully demonstrated this same principle, spontaneously, to the seminarians. Whenever you want any hypnotic results with your patients, you had better mean what you say. All you need to do [in order to convince yourself] is to look back through your own personal history as a functioning human being. Look back to when you've had an anesthesia, when you've had analgesia. Recognize that you've had amnesia for pain on innumerable occasions. You really don't differ from other, normal human beings. Your total experience should teach you that you are not asking anything of your patients that is beyond their abilities. When you give a suggestion to a patient, you'd better keep in mind, "I *know* this patient can develop an analgesia—I *know* this patient can develop an anesthesia—I *know* this patient can develop amnesia."

Structured Amnesias

There is another factor involved in developing anesthesia or analgesia or amnesia. When a patient comes into my office [for a scheduled appointment], I usually have a rather clear idea of what I want to do. If I think that it would be a good idea for this patient to leave my office with an amnesia for everything that happens during the hour—if that is my clinical judgment—what do I do?

125

As the patient enters my office I say, "Is there much traffic outside today? Was there much traffic on North Central Avenue? How warm is it—I haven't had a chance to get outside today?" And I ask a few other questions about what he has seen or noticed on the way to the office.

The patient answers all the questions. He sits down; the session takes place; he gets up to leave, and I say, "North Central Avenue really wasn't crowded today." I reorient the patient back to the same topic I had discussed at the beginning of the session—as if nothing whatsover had intervened. In other words, I step backward to the initial conversation so that the patient walks out thinking about North Central Avenue, about the temperature, the amount of traffic, the mocking birds in the trees, and *not* about what happened in the office. Thus the patient may very often leave the session with an amnesia for it.

Indirect Approaches to Analgesia: Associating Pleasure and Pain

When I want a patient to develop an analgesia I am quite willing first to let him tell me all about his pain until I can see from the expression on his face that he knows I understand. And I'm not averse to making a few remarks to indicate that I *do* understand. Then I might ask the patient some simple question that inadvertently takes him far away from this matter of pain. Suppose, for example, that his pain developed during the last hot day we had had; and that last hot day occurred sometime during last month; and last month was just this past winter. I will then switch far from the matter of winter and ask, "Where did you spend last summer?"

Now, the patient might be rather surprised at such a question, but it doesn't take very long to get him going on the matter of last summer. Last summer he had not had that pain. So we go into the question of the pleasures and joys and satisfactions of last summer. I emphasize comfort, physical ease, joys, and satisfactions, and I point out how nice it is to continue to remember the joys and satisfactions of last summer; the physical ease of last summer. If the patient seems to be getting a bit edgy, I remind him of the time "when you were rowing the boat, and you got that blister on your hand, and it hurt quite a bit, but fortunately, it healed up." [What am I doing?] I am not afraid to mention hurt or pain or distress, but I mention it far away from that backache the patient brought to the session. I mentioned a pain from a blister from rowing a boat last summer, and I haven't been shocked by that uneasy expression on his face.

In hypnosis your task is to guide patients' thinking, to guide the association of ideas along channels that are therapeutic. You know very, very well that you can have a painful spot in your leg and yet you can forget all about that painful spot on your leg, or the pain in your arm, or that aching tooth, by simply losing yourself in a suspenseful movie; by losing yourself in the action on the screen.

If you are operating on a patient in your office and you know that it can cause pain, you should also know that you can direct your patient's thinking to an area far removed from that pain situation.

I am thinking of a patient who said to me, "I'm so afraid to go to the dentist—I agonize so much and perspire so frightfully that I'm in absolute misery!"

I asked that patient immediately, "Did you do that as a child? What was your favorite sport as a child?"

"Did you do that as a child?" was a completely fearless question. I was listening to this patient's complaint about pain, anxiety, distress, and suddenly I asked her what she did in her childhood. I began by talking about her *anxiety,* and she knew it, and then I asked her what her favorite *pleasure* was as a child. How do you get from pain, anxiety, and distress to *pleasure as a child?* Good question.

She promptly told me about her favorite pleasure as a child, and she was delighted to talk about that pleasure because the matter of the dental office concerned fear and anxiety and distress, and it was so much more delightful to discuss with me that favorite activity from her childhood. I tied the two issues of pain and pleasure together by the immediate succession of questions: "Did you have those anxieties as a child?"—and—"What was your favorite sport?"

Since she had told me about all her favorite pleasures as a

child, and about one pleasure in particular, I suggested to her that when she went to the dentist's office, that as she settled down in that dental chair, as she really squirmed around in the chair and really felt her seat on the chair seat, really felt her back on the back of the chair, her arms on the arms of the chair, and her head on the headrest, that *she would have an overwhelming recollection of her favorite childhood activity which would absolutely dominate the entire situation.*

What had I done? I brought up the realities of the dental chair—squirming around to get a comfortable seat, feeling the back of the dental chair, feeling the arms of the dental chair—and I even wriggled around the way I wanted her to do in that dental chair. Then as soon as she had settled all the squirming, I told her to move herself back into the memories of her favorite childhood activity. Her favorite activity had been playing in the leaves on the lawn. In the autumn you can build great big houses out of the leaves, nice pathways through piles of leaves; you can jump in the leaves, you can bury yourself in the leaves, you can throw the leaves all around you.

And so she simply went into a very, very nice, anesthetic trance state. Now and then the dentist would ask her some stupid question when all she really wanted to do was to think about those leaves. She would notice mentally that here was some stupid person trying to talk to her while she was very busy burying herself in the leaves; probably some grown-up yelling at her, but she was too interested in the leaves to give much notice. She could have dental surgery performed. The dentist thought she was a most cooperative patient.

What was your favorite activity as a child? I could really get my patient to elaborate on that subject. In other words, you very carefully raise a question in such a way that you slide past the difficulty—past the problem the patient is dealing with—and start up another train of mental activity, of emotional activity, that precludes the possibility of feeling pain. My sophisticated subjects—those with training in clinical psychology and those who are themselves psychiatrists—will first pick apart the technique I have used on them, and will then proceed to recognize the validity of it from their own experience. And they will have me employ precisely the same techniques on them again, because they know that they are human, and that they can do the same thing with pleasure, over and over again.

I think it is an error to strive for an anesthesia or an analgesia by direct methods alone. I think you should be willing to bring either phenomenon about indirectly. Every time you tell a patient, "Forget that this is a watch," you are asking that person to do a specific thing—to forget—to forget what?—a watch! Now, remember, forget the watch! That's what you are saying when you say, "Forget the watch." [You are actually giving a negative suggestion to remember the watch.]

But you can ask the patient to look at this watch, an interesting thing. It rather amuses me. It's rather fascinating how you can look at something and become tremendously fascinated with just looking at it, and then the topic of conversation changes and you drift far away to that trip you took in Europe. Now, what was it I came up here for? And you drift far, far away from that watch, because you start following your own trains of thought.

Altered Reality in Symptom Relief

The next matter that you should bear in mind about your patient is that when you take away the sense of feeling through hypnotic anesthesia, or you bring about an analgesia, you have asked your patient to make an entirely different kind of reality orientation. Earlier today I mentioned that experiment wherein I asked unsuspecting students to discover what mental processes were involved in picking up an imaginary apple and putting it on a real table in front of them. Just what were those mental processes? A goodly number of the students complained of feeling funny all over and left that situation without finishing it. They were losing their contact with reality. Therefore they felt "funny."

Now, when you induce an analgesia you are asking your patient to lose a certain amount of his reality contact. You are asking him to alter it. Then he begins to feel funny, which he may or may not recognize. But he can react to that funny feeling by getting out of the situation, because it is a strange situation for him. Therefore, whenever you induce an analgesia or an anesthesia, you see to it that your patient doesn't get frightened by his altered reality orientation. I let those students feel funny all over and I let them run out on me because their spontaneous responses were an important experimental finding that I wanted to study. I could afford to let them run out. But when you are working with patients in your office and they get those funny feelings, they want to run out too! They may not know why; they may not know it's because of the funny feelings; but they *do* know they want to leave. But they can't afford to leave, and you can't afford to let them leave.

That is why it is your obligation to tell them that one of the astonishing things is that as they begin to feel more and more comfortable, or as they get more and more interested in this or that, perhaps they will notice that the light in the office is of a softer hue. Quite often I have told patients, "I hope you don't mind, but as we continue our work here in the office the light will automatically dim and become softer, or become lighter."

I had one patient who experienced that dimming of the light and that increasing of the light. He couldn't understand how it happened because he had checked all the switches in the office and did not find any doo-hickey on them to cause that fluctuation in the light. He wondered if I had a secret control somewhere. His reality orientation had been disturbed. I had told him already that it was fine if the lights changed, and so he felt reassured; and being trained in electrical matters, he immediately interpreted that change as caused by something within his experience with which he was familiar [an electrical attachment of some kind]. So although he misinterpreted the cause, it was still acceptable to his orientation.

Then there are patients who tell me that the office is getting lighter or darker, warmer or colder, bigger or smaller; that they feel taller or shorter, more relaxed or more afraid, more alert or more sluggish. All manner of changes in one's sense of reality are possible in hypnosis. Whenever you want to elicit anesthesia or analgesia be very careful not to suggest a specific focus. Instead, note the patient's reaction carefully so that you can then

130

offer a casual statement based on that reaction. I had one patient who worked for General Electric. I noticed his reaction and thought it might be a pupillary response to the thought, *the office is getting darker.* So, I made the simple comment that possibly a bulb had blown out. The patient looked satisfied and pleased with that explanation and I did not have to disturb his trance any further. A bulb does blow out now and then. There is nothing unusual or remarkable about that. But I was attentive to my patient's response [so that I could utilize that response to help maintain his trance].

Trance Deepening and the Patient's World View

Next, I want to discuss this matter of trance deepening. It is most difficult to deepen trances when the patients prefer light trance states, and when they do not realize that different trance depths can be learned. I have patients who insist on remaining in very light trances. I'd better go along with them and never try to deepen their trances. It is my obligation—my duty—not to try to deepen those trances, because as surely as I try to deepen those trances, and the patients recognize that I am trying, then I am violating their personal understandings of what is right and good. Patients will come into your office with their concepts of hypnosis such that they expect exceedingly light trances. I think you had better be willing to work with that, and you'd better be willing to praise patients for being able to accomplish so much in so light a trance.

I think also you ought to be willing to express some doubt to patients as to whether they are really in a trance state, because "it seems too light to be really a trance state." The effect of saying this usually is to deepen the trance. But the question is, are you being honest with your patients by deceiving them in this regard? I think so. Patients come to you for medical or dental help. They do not come to you for scientific instruction on trance levels. Patients aren't the least bit interested in the philosophical approach to hypnosis. They are interested in medical or dental hypnosis. They want certain personal results, but their knowledge of the language is such that they are handicapped.

131

Therefore, you'd better be willing to use the language that patients understand: If they understand that a very light trance is the right thing, you go ahead and call a very deep trance a very light trance; and in that very deep trance you had better see to it that they have evidence somewhere that they are in a very light trance. In this regard it is a rather simple matter to drop a pencil on the floor so that patients take notice—after which you comment that they really aren't in too *deep* a trance, and that you would like them to remain at that *depth* of trance. Patients don't recognize that you are saying *depth*. You don't tell them to stay at the same *lightness* of trance, but you give them simple, ordinary clues in the language that they understand: "You really aren't in too *deep* a trance." Whenever you fight with patients, whenever you try to force patients to do things your way, you end up on the losing side of the deal.

Accepting and Utilizing the Patient's Point of View

I am thinking of a patient I saw for Dr. Pearson. The gentleman said to me, "I want you to hypnotize me," meanwhile giving me a very, very cold shoulder in body language. I acted as if I believed he actually wanted me to hypnotize him. That patient was not aware of his own unconscious resistances.

When I asked, "Do you want me to hypnotize you in a light trance, a medium trance, or a deep trance?", he crossed his legs and brought his hands way over to the side—drawing himself even further away from me—and answered simply that he thought a deep trance would be the better trance! Well, I could see the real meaning of that behavior. I acted as if I believed every word that man had said, but I also knew that he would not be able to go into a trance. My task was to get him to recognize that what he really needed was not a trance but some psychiatric help. When I initiated this topic he immediately turned around to face me squarely and proceeded to talk about his need for psychiatric help. We discussed the various issues—just what a psychiatric interview would involve, for instance; not what a psychiatric interview would involve *for him,* but what a psychiatric interview was *in general.*

132

Similarly, when you discuss a deep trance with a patient, *whose* deep trance is the issue? You don't discuss Joe Blow's deep trance, or Aunt Betsy's deep trance. You discuss *deep trance* in general. That way the patient can wonder, *He is talking about a deep trance, and I wonder if I want a deep trance.*

You have labelled deep trance as one possibility, medium trance as another possibility, and light trance still another. And then you wind up having each person experience the trance state that best fits the individual personality. Your success rests on the patient's own ability to reconcile each point you mention with his own unconscious understandings. I always ask my patient to exercise his own best level of understanding, because he had better understand. It is his own best level of understanding that he will have to employ if he is going to achieve any benefits.

You tell the patient, "You want to go into a trance; you want to achieve certain results. You don't know whether it's a light trance, a deep trance, or a medium trance that you want, and neither do I. I think you and I ought to let your unconscious mind use whatever amount of light trance, whatever amount of medium trance, and whatever amount of deep trance that your unconscious naturally feels will be most helpful."

You verbalize these ideas in such a way that your patient can understand them and be free to accept them. The patient is free to deepen his trance; he is free to come up into a light trance or to a medium trance, and to go back down into a deep trance. I think too many practitioners are distressed when their patient comes out of a deep trance and slides into a light trance to look around and see what on earth you are up to now. I think you ought to be pleased when your patient does that, because he is looking around to see what you are doing. He is taking a good, comprehensive look, and I doubt that there is anything negative about that. Now, perhaps, the patient can understand the situation even better, so that his unconscious can carry out the hypnotic goals still further.

Why shouldn't a patient engage in that type of behavior? He has come out of his deep trance to look around to see if additional factors have arisen, for he has lost a good deal of his reality orientation by going into that deep trance. Several of my friends who are anesthesiologists have told me of instances in which a patient in a deep, hypnotic anesthesia suddenly comes out of the anesthesia to look around and see what's happening. The proper handling of this behavior is simply to say, "Now that you've looked around and oriented yourself, you can go right back into that very deep trance." Some anesthesiologists do get frightened and upset the first time a patient comes out of hypnoanesthesia in mid-operation. But often, when handled properly, the patient can achieve even better hypnotic results after his brief period of re-orientation.

QUESTIONS AND ANSWERS

The Patient's Special Knowledge

Q. In the treatment of pain and symptoms you implied that anything we know as doctors about the physiology of the patient from an anatomical, neurological, or functional standpoint should be communicated to the patient before we attempt to carry out hypnotic work. Is that correct?

A: Anything that stands out psychologically, neurologically, or physically we really ought to take into consideration first and then give patients whatever knowledge they need to have along those lines. They don't need to have too much information, but they may need to understand some details about muscle feeling, or nerve pathways, or whatever.

Q: Can patients also tell us many things about themselves that we cannot observe, and that we might not elicit by normal interview techniques?

A: Patients can often tell you things that are utterly surprising. I had a topic to explain to a psychology class. I looked

134

at a particular member of the psychology class and I immediately asked, "Are you willing to act as a volunteer?" She said that she was willing.

"Do you mind leaving the room? I want to speak to the rest of the class."

She left the room and in her absence I told the class: "Watch that girl. She is going to go into a trance and she is going to describe the trance to you in tactile terms—in terms of touch, in terms of kinesthetic sensations, in terms of body sensations. I know this because I could tell by looking at her that she is a girl that *feels*."

So the class watched her go into a trance. They didn't notice anything particular in her behavior, but for me it was a very delightful thing to watch her in that trance. The class knew that I had never seen this girl before. When she came out of the trance and I asked her to describe what it had been like for her, her reply was rather astonishing:

"The first thing I noticed was that the soles of my feet changed . . .", and she proceeded to describe how her hypnosis had developed from the soles of her feet upward. I asked her to describe the changes more specifically.

"You know, I became awfully aware of my fistula, and I could feel parastalsis, and then when I swallowed I could trace that swallow all the way down to my stomach. I could feel my heart beating, and I could feel muscle movements inside my chest with every breath."

She was one of these feeling people. The class sat there bug-eyed, watching her and listening to her describe those feeling sensations. She described how she felt her jaw lose all sensation, how she felt her upper lip lose all sensation, and then how she finally lost contact with her scalp. Where was she then? Her statement was, "I was a listening entity willing to do whatever you suggested, but I had no body." She had lost all contact with her body. Now that was a most delightful and utterly instructive statement for me to hear. You always ask patients to give you some of the highlights of their trance developments.

135

The Double Bind: Illusory Choice to Bypass Resistance, Facilitate Rapport and Unexpected Trance, and Achieve Symptom Relief

I need subjects in order to demonstrate. The best kind of subjects to use for demonstrations are, of course, strangers. The kind of situation I want to demonstrate right now requires a subject who has not volunteered to be a subject, who does not expect to be a subject, and who is not the least bit interested in being a subject. Why? Because that is most often the situation with patients who come into your office for hypnosis: they do not expect to have hypnosis used, they are not particularly interested in it, and it takes them entirely by surprise.

Now, this is what I would like to do. There happens to be a young lady sitting in the audience over there who is wearing a very white hat with a veil on it.

"Mrs. Linden, will you please go over and take that young lady by the right hand—not by the left hand, but by the right hand—and bring her up here?"

What I want to demonstrate to you is this: In the use of hypnosis for anesthesia, for dentistry, even for interpersonal relations, there is this matter called the double bind.

[To the subject with the white hat,] "You have already demonstrated what I wanted you to demonstrate."

This woman declared that she did not want to come up here. The gentleman next to her stated that she had declined. But I asked Mrs. Linden here to go over and get the girl wearing the white hat with the veil on it and to be *sure* to bring her up on stage by taking her by the *right* hand. Mrs. Linden went over. Now, this young lady could not refuse to come up here because I didn't actually *ask* her. She couldn't refuse Mrs. Linden because Mrs. Linden did not *ask* her. Nobody had actually *asked* her to come up. I had simply asked Mrs. Linden to take the subject by her right hand and lead her up; but I didn't *ask* her to come. This is awfully important because when you *ask* patients to do something you are also giving them the opportunity of *refusing*. So, you ask something in such a way that they can't possibly refuse. My subject was awfully angry on her way up. I had hoped that she would refuse to come up here because that would have made things even more informative.

You can approach patients in the same way you approach children. How do you ask your children to go to bed? Do you say emphatically, "It's eight o'clock, time to go to bed!" If you do, you probably get a lot of refusals! Why not ask instead, "Would you like to go to bed at a quarter to eight, or at eight o'clock?" Every normal child will respond immediately, "At eight o'clock, not at a quarter to eight!" And so it is with your patients.

In this matter of using hypnosis for dental anesthesia, ask your patients, "Do you want it to hurt *a lot,* or *a little? Do you want the hypnosis to remove *all of the pain,* or do you want the hypnosis to leave *a little bit of the pain?"* And patients will tell you they want the hypnosis to relieve *all of the pain.* What have they told you? They have told you that they want hypnosis, and they have told you the purpose for using the hypnosis. The important thing is that *they tell you.*

I frequently use the double bind in questioning patients: "Do you want to get over your bad habit this week or next week? But that length of time doesn't really seem reasonable to me. Wouldn't you rather take a more reasonable length of time to get over your habit, such as three weeks?"

What have I really asked them? I have asked them to specify the length of time that they are going to need to get over a habit. I haven't asked them, *"Are you going to get over the habit?"* I haven't asked them to decide that important question. I merely ask them to choose the length of time, but *implicit in their choice of one week or two weeks or three weeks is the assumption that they are going to get over their habit.*

A patient comes into my office and says, "I simply cannot tell you my story."

I say, "There is no particular hurry about telling it to me today. If you prefer, tell it to me during our next appointment, or two appointments later."

And so the patient can tell me his story either during our next appointment or two appointments later, but *he is going to tell me his story.* You see, in this matter of communicating with

137

patients, it is tremendously important to give them the opportunity of cooperating with you [rather than forcing them to decide these matters alone]. It is rather venturesome and rather frightening for patients to make decisive statements about their situations. They want desperately to have things come out in the right way, and naturally they don't want to decide immediately on something that is so terribly difficult.

FIRST DEMONSTRATION

The Double Bind to Facilitate Trance*

[Erickson now talks directly to the subject with the white hat whose name is June.]

Erickson (E): Now, tell me what happened. How is your heart rate?

June (J): Better.

E: I am glad of that. Would you like to get even with Mrs. Linden?

J: Yes.

E: Do you think you could take her by the left hand and bring her up here? [Pause as subject brings Mrs. L up on stage.] Now, which one of you ought to be in a trance *first*?

Now, I am again using a double bind. I've asked who should be in a trance *first*. This matter is between them (an argument). I am out here in front where everything is safe. Actually, I think that they are both good subjects.

*See *Collected Papers,* Vol. I, for an extensive presentation of the various forms of the double bind.

J: Otherwise I wouldn't be up here!

E: I didn't really inquire about that. Now, let's go into that double bind. Mrs. Linden says that June should go into a trance first, and June says, "Well, I am a good subject." But Mrs. Linden, what does it mean when you say June should go *first*—then who goes *second?*

Mrs. L: I didn't figure that right. [Laughter]

E: But there is the double bind for Mrs. Linden, as well as for June. Now they have *both* agreed to be hypnotic subjects. [To June] Do you ordinarily go into a trance standing up? Is it easier standing up?

J: I have never tried it standing up.

E: How many of you recognize the double bind right there? [To June] You didn't want to go into a trance a few minutes ago, did you?

J: No.

E: "A few minutes ago you didn't want to go into a trance" means what? Now you *do* want to go into a trance—the double bind again!

Mrs. L: You get her coming and going.

E: That's what I mean. I have been perfectly courteous to both of you, haven't I?

J and Mrs. L: Yes.

I have been courteous. I have been using them to illustrate my point, but nevertheless, in presenting ideas to you and to them, I have built up a situation in which they have to give cooperative answers.

Questions to Facilitate Difficult
Medical and Dental Problems

What do you want to achieve with your patient who desperately needs medical care or dental care and yet is fearful and anxious and unable to decide to get that care? You ought to be able to ask important questions in such a way that the patient has a comfortable feeling about giving the proper answer; so that he does not have to confront himself with that horrible statement: "Yes, I need an amputation at the knee joint—go ahead and amputate my leg!" That is an awfully hard statement for any patient to make. You know that he has a carcinoma of the ankle. You know that the amputation should be done. You ought to be willing to put the question to the patient in such a way that the patient can agree to the amputation without feeling, "I went in and told that doctor to cut off my leg." That's a horrible thing for most patients to be confronted with. And I do have patients who tell me that they have had that kind of experience.

[Erickson again addresses the two subjects.]

E: I would really like to use you as hypnotic subjects. This time I will simply ask you directly. Personally, would you like to try to go into a trance? I do have other subjects.

J: I would rather not.

E: How about you, Mrs. Linden?

Mrs. L: I would rather not.

E: Thank you both for a very competent demonstration.

When Dr. Kubie was co-authoring various articles with me we discussed at length these matters of permissiveness, of authoritative approach, and of illusory freedom of choice. Patients who go into a dental office or a medical office are there out of necessity. They really do not have a choice. They have cavities, or they have abscesses, or they have stomach ulcers, or whatever. They are there because of an absolute necessity. Yet nobody likes to feel compelled. Patients are hesitant and fearful and uncertain about their own reactions. You ought to be willing to learn how to talk to patients so that you can give them what Kubie has termed "illusory freedom of choice." Of course, you must be the final judge of what is the adequate medical or dental care to be given, but patients really ought to feel as comfortable as possible.

Misusing the Double Bind

You know patients' needs. You ought to help patients make their own proper decisions, and you ought to make those decisions as easy as possible for patients to make. This brings us to the matter of using the double bind for your own selfish purposes. I know of some doctors who ask patients, "Do you want to pay your bill this week, or next week?" Patients unconsciously recognize the double bind and so decide, "I'll pay the bill this week, and find someone else to go to next week!" In other words, the use of the double bind has to be in favor of the patient, never in favor of yourself.

In the use of hypnosis the very generosity of your attitude allows patients to feel utterly comfortable. Now I'm perfectly willing to put my patients in the double bind, but they also sense unconsciously that I will never, never, hold them to it. They know that I will yield anytime; they know that I will put them in a different double bind in some other situation so that they can make use of that new and different double bind that meets their needs more adequately. If you ever use the double bind selfishly, you will undoubtedly lose patients.

[Erickson addresses the two subjects still on stage.]

E: **How do you feel about** *my selfish use of you for the benefit of the group?*

141

J: I didn't think it was selfish.

E: Did you recognize that I put you in a double bind just now? I did! If you had said that you didn't like my use of you then you also would have been saying that this group is not entitled to the benefit of this demonstration—and you'd be caught!

Practical Applications of the Double Bind: Allen's Hundred Stitches

I hope you really don't mind my willingness to define these issues clearly, because in all of your contacts you ought to practice a double bind; you ought to learn thoroughly how to apply it in all kinds of different situations. I am thinking about an example I published in *The American Journal of Clinical Hypnosis.* Many years ago my eight-year-old son, Allen, was running across a vacant lot when suddenly he fell down on a broken bottle which split the front of his leg horribly. We had nicknamed Allen, "The Noise," because you could always tell where he was simply by listening. Sure enough, he now came roaring into the house, roaring at the top of his voice, with blood streaming down his leg.

Now, what could I do for a screaming eight-year-old boy who was obviously in pain and obviously frightened; who was badly injured and bleeding profusely? As he came charging into the house, I took one quick look and yelled, "Use the bath towel, not the hand towel!—the bath towel, not the hand towel!—*the bath towel,* not the hand towel!" Now Allen wasn't using *any* towel, but I seemed to want him to use a bath towel, and so he was caught between the hand towel and the bath towel—but he *was* using a towel. By that time someone had brought a bath towel to me and I handed it to Allen, saying, "Wrap it up this way, not that way—*this way* ... tighter, not so tight ... tighter, not so tight!" A double bind again.

All the way to the surgeon's office I kept insisting to Allen that he be sure that the surgeon allow Allen his full surgical rights: "Don't let that doctor do the wrong thing. Be sure that he puts in as many stitches as possible. Your sister is always bragging about her fifty stitches, so don't let that doctor put in less than fifty stitches. You are entitled to as many stitches as Betty Alice got!"

Allen proceeded to rehearse his demands mentally and verbally in the car. As we walked into the surgeon's office the receptionist looked at the bloody towel and said, "This way, please," to which Allen immediately replied, "I want a hundred stitches!"

She didn't know what to think, but she took us into the surgery room whereupon Allen yelled at the surgeon, *"I want a hundred stitches!"* Then, as the injury was being sponged and cleaned and sewed up Allen continued to protest, "You're putting those stitches too far apart!" And the surgeon kept looking up at me, and looking down at Allen, looking up at me. Allen was caught there. He wanted a hundred stitches. Here was a surgeon who obviously wasn't going to oblige. But Allen knew his rights and so he kept yelling, "More stitches, closer together—put more stitches in there—there's room to put one more stitch in between those two!" And Allen protested all the way home because Betty Alice had the lead in the number of stitches.

Here was the double bind: "Use the bath towel, not the hand towel"—Allen wasn't using either; "Be sure you get as many stitches as possible"—when really he didn't want *any* stitches. And where did Allen's anesthesia come from? I didn't have to tell him not to have pain. There was no need for that. Allen was very, very, busy on this tremendously important project of getting more stitches than his sister had had. Allen wasn't expecting pain; he wasn't interested in pain; he was interested in his full surgical rights. Now I kept telling him, "Don't let that surgeon talk you out of it—you really ought to see if you can't get a hundred stitches!"

Allen still remembers that episode with the greatest of pleasure. He is a mathematician at the present time, and he is trying to figure out a mathematical formula to explain what on earth happened to that pain sensation.

SECOND DEMONSTRATION

Relaxation in Hypnosis

E: [To subject already on stage] Now, I really don't know anything about you, your hypnotic history, or what you've learned.

But one of the important things that everyone here today has learned is the importance of having a subject relax. But just what do you mean by relaxation? Do you mean that patients must lie down on a couch and relax all the muscles of their bodies; or do you mean that they can have a general, relaxed attitude? When the Captain says, "At ease!", to the Private he is literally telling the Private, "Relax." Now, as the subject stands here she is going to be alert and attentive, and she is going to demonstrate that she is not in a trance right now. And you can watch her body mobility and see that she is not in a trance.

E: Now, you've never seen me induce a trance. How do you think I go about it?

S: [I don't know.]*

E: You really don't know. Do you suppose there is any important thing to do about inducing a trance?

S: [Well, maybe a light touch to my hand or arm?]

E: So you think there should be physical contact. Now, one of the things that we all learn from childhood is that it is possible to communicate by a nod of the head, by turning the head from side to side. Do you recognize that you *may* be in a light trance? Do you suppose you can go even more deeply into a

---

*Subject responses are bracketed to indicate the presumed response when actual response was lost in the recording.

light trance? And just let your hand slowly touch your face, and take a deep breath, and go much more deeply into a trance. That's right, just close your eyes.

Individual Meanings in Eyelid Fluttering

Of course, catalepsy is present; there seems to be catalepsy in her one arm.

One of the things that often troubles the beginner in hypnosis, and also often troubles operators who have had experiences in hypnosis, is the eye flutter. The eyelids flutter. I have noticed that happening in subjects from time to time over the years. I've found that you can demonstrate the most profound anesthesia in subjects who have a fluttering of the eyelids; in other subjects, there will be a fluttering of the eyelids synonymous with the light trance; in still others you get fluttering of the eyelids as synonymous with the medium trance. You never really know what fluttering of the eyelids means from one patient to another. But it does have a meaning for each patient.

If you are disturbed by it, the patient will also be disturbed about it. If you're not disturbed about it, the patient isn't going to be either. If you see an expression of anxiety on the patient's face you ought to tell that patient that the fluttering of the eyelids is perfectly all right.

Dissocation in the Light Trance

E: Now, why did you open your eyes and rouse up?

S: [I don't know.]

E: You really don't know, do you? In what way did I touch your elbow differently?

S: [I just felt I should open my eyes.]

E: You felt you should open your eyes. Now, why did your

arm go up? [Pause as the subject remains silent] You have no answer. Are you awake right now?

S: [I think so.]

E: You think you are. Are you sure about that?

S: [Yes.]

E: Why? Do you think that everybody else agrees that you are awake? Is it customary in your area to keep your hand up?

S: No.

E: When you are awake, you keep your hand down here, right?

S: Yes.

E: And are you awake right now?

Here is the lady who goes into a light trance. She is illustrating a point that I think all of you ought to keep in mind. She can verbalize slightly, but her hands and her arms seem to be apart from her. She is illustrating dissociation of a part of her body. In dentistry, you want this part of the body dissociated; in surgery of the leg, you want that part dissociated. Why do you always need a complete, somnambulistic trance when you can bring about a dissociation of a part of the body in a light trance? Marjorie, the lady in the blue dress at the Orthodontic Association Meeting this morning, had said that her arm was another entity entirely.

E: Do you agree with Marjorie?

S: Yes. It feels like it isn't connected.

E: That it isn't connected.

I've had subjects in deep trances, in light trances, in medium trances, subjects in their first trances—all speak spontaneously about this "disconnection" they have experienced. The psychologically trained person is very likely to describe the feeling as a "dissociation." The person not trained in psychological or psychiatric thinking is very likely to use the term "disconnected." It does feel that way.

Delicate Tactile Guidance for Dissociation and Trance Awakening

E: You don't know why you opened your eyes before.

S: I think I opened them by the touch of the elbow.

E: By the touch of the elbow.

Now, this is the next point that I want to establish with you. You all saw her standing there with her eyes closed when suddenly she opened them. Why? She didn't know, and I asked her about touching her elbow, and gave her a chance to think.

E: And I did touch your elbow differently, didn't I?

S: Yes, as if you wanted me . . . [Pause]

E: As if I wanted you to what?

S: To wake up.

E: You see? When I want a subject to develop disconnection of the arm I am very likely to touch it very, very gently. I suggest by the touch the direction in which I want the hand to move, and when I want to rouse . . .

S: It's a firmer touch.

E: It's a different kind of touch, and she opened her eyes,

saying, "What's going on here?—this is a different kind of approach!" Are you used to facing an audience like this?

S: No, but I am not uncomfortable.

E: Thank you very much.

E: [To new subject] I have worked with you before, haven't I? How do you ordinarily go into a trance?

S: I close my eyes.

E: You just close your eyes and relax. Have you ever gone into a trance without closing your eyes?

S: No.

E: Why not?

S: I don't know, I just never have.

E: You have never even tried, have you?

S: No.

E: Have you looked at your hand with your eyes open to go into a trance? [Pause] Well, look at your hand, and keep right on looking.
[Turning to another new subject] Now, I have said you could nod your head, you could turn it from side to side. Have you ever gone into a trance with your eyes open? [Quietly and expectantly] Are you in a trance right now?

S: I don't know.

E: [Quietly] You don't know, that's right. Now, is it really important for you to know whether you are or are not in a trance?

Trance Validity without Patient Awareness

Recognize that there are many medical and dental men who think it is awfully important that patients know whether or not they are in trances. And it really isn't important. Very often, my patients don't even know that they are in trances. Similarly, in lecturing to a group of psychology students, certain students noticed from time to time that *other* members of the class were in trances, but they didn't notice that those other members were noticing that *they* were in trances. At the end of a lecture hour I asked the group as a whole whether any of them had ever been in trances. I got a very nice, negative answer from the entire group. Then one half of the class looked in astonishment at the other half of the class, and vice versa, because each half had been noticing the other half go into trances! So why is it important for subjects or patients to know that they are in trances?

Body Movement and Time Distortion in Light Trance

E: In what connection have you experienced hypnosis before—in dental or medical work?

S: In dental work.

E: How do you suppose you would figure out whether or not you had been in a trance? Are you interested in figuring it out?

S: Yes.

Now, if those of you in the audience will study other members of the audience for a moment you will notice that there is a lot of head movement, shoulder movement, and body adjusting that you don't see happening in this subject. [This means the subject is in a light trance already. His attention is so focused on me that his normal body movements are subsiding.]

In a psychology class situation I stand there courteously, patiently, and I wait and wait and wait until finally it dawns on the class what I am doing. I am waiting for them to quiet down and focus their attention on me. [They can learn better that way.]

In these types of situations you also can discover the phenomenon of time distortion. Even subjects in such a light trance as this subject is in, [with the subtle slowing down of head and body movements], will show a changed appreciation and alteration in their sense of time. Now, of course I have been talking to the audience, but my subject has been able to hear me, and so I have spoiled the experimental situation.

Permission for Trance: Verbal (Explicit) Versus Nonverbal (Implicit) Behavior

E: Dr. S. tells me that you have been trained not to go into a trance until you have first given your verbal permission. I didn't ask your verbal permission, did I? Do you think you are in a trance? Is it distressing, this situation of uncertainty on your part?

S: Not particularly—just a little.

E: Now what is verbal permission? Is it the formal pronouncement of certain words, or is it the implications of your behavior? Verbal permission could be a nod of your head because that nod would be understood as a yes, isn't that right? Or, if I asked you to stand up and go into a trance, and you stood up, that would be permission, right? Do you feel better now? You recognize that you are in a trance. Your response is different—it lacks that tone of anxiety. Tell me, do you ordinarily hold your hand like that? How does your arm feel?

S: It's all right. Feels comfortable.

E: All right, close your eyes, take a deep breath, and go deeper asleep. Now I don't know whether you have been taught

150

hypnosis by the use of the word *deeper* or the word *trance,* but there is no question of your ability to understand correctly the meaning of my utterances.

Preliminary Understanding to Cover Verbal Mistakes

And so it is in dealing with patients. The careful worker says to the patient, "Now, there are certain goals and objectives that we have fairly well in mind as we work together. If I express something inadequately or incorrectly, try to understand the correct meaning. And when you do not fully express yourself, I, too, will do my best to understand you."

I stress this point for the following reason. When talking to patients, we very often make slips of the tongue—we say the wrong thing, and then go into a panic because we have said the wrong thing to the patient. You yourself ought to have the attitude that you are definitely human, you are subject to error, and that sometimes you are bound to speak incorrectly. Then you should establish this as a preliminary understanding with the patient, stressing that you are working toward a very definite and common goal: "If I happen to say, 'Wake up,' when I mean, 'Sleep deeper,' you will understand, because I'm thinking of many things and I might misspeak." You really ought to have this kind of understanding with patients so that you don't go into a panic when you make a slip of the tongue or when you say the wrong thing; so that you don't get flustered when you get a bit incoherent because you are shifting trains of thought in the suggestions you are offering. After all, those suggestions are merely a means of keeping contact.

Implicit Versus Explicit Meaning: Sharing as a Corrective Emotional Experience

E: By the way, what are you thinking about?

S: I'm listening to you.

E: Do you think I am speaking very accurately?

S: I think so.

E: Do you agree with me? All right. Now take a deep breath and open your eyes and awaken wide awake.

Now first I had asked this subject to take a deep breath, close her eyes and go deep asleep; and now I just asked her to take a deep breath and open her eyes and awaken. In other words, it isn't what you say at a given moment that is important; it is the meaning that you are conveying. Therefore, it is awfully important for you to be aware of the meanings you want to convey. You ought to study your words; you ought to learn to recognize all the possible meanings in them.

For example, Dr. Steingart had an experience in which he asked his subject to regress to a happy experience from her past that she would be willing to share with the audience. To his distress and horror, she regressed to a traumatic experience. Now this was rather disturbing to the audience, rather distressing to him, but apparently it was not particularly distressing to the subject.

I pointed out to Dr. Steingart the meaning of his wording to "regress to some previous experience—a happy one—that you are willing to *share* with others." He asked for a happy experience. Now what is it that we all wish for in regard to a sad, unhappy experience? We wish it were a happy one. We want it to be an exprience that we can *share* with others. Therefore, if we can share it with others that proves it is a happy thing. You certainly aren't going to share a miserable, unhappy event with other people. You feel, naturally, that it is your own misfortune and you are not going to thrust it on others, and anything you are willing to give to others is going to be pleasant. So, *the process of sharing an unhappy experience is a corrective measure.* Dr. Steingart said that the damage seemed to have been suffered by the audience and himself, and that the subject herself did not show any particular signs of distress. Sharing is awfully important, and you ought to know the meaning of your words.

Questioning with Conviction to Indirectly Facilitate Regression and Hallucination

E: Now, I think I will turn to the lady in the blue dress. What did I do with you last year?

S: I don't remember.

E: You don't remember. It was very interesting. I remember, and you were in this room, and you were standing right there! You may sit down—go ahead. You really can't remember last year at all?

S: I haven't thought about it.

E: You haven't thought about it. Let's see. Who was sitting there, do you remember? That's it. What year is it?

S: It is 1961. [It is actually 1962.]

E: And you don't know who that person is? [Subject shakes head.] No, you don't know. I am going to ask you this same question next year around May 2, 1962. Will that be all right? And what is the answer you are going to give me?

S: I don't know.

E: You don't know. All right, close your eyes.

What did I ask of this subject? I started talking about last year—did she remember this or that; had she stood here in this same position. She hadn't thought about it, frankly speaking. Whenever you ask a question of a person [to facilitate development of various hypnotic phenomena] you really ought to ask that question as if you meant it. When I question a patient, I mean that question that I ask, and I am utterly sincere. When I asked this subject today if she knew that person sitting there [where there was no actual person], I truly meant that person sitting right there—not here, not over there, but *right*

153

there; and so she looked and she didn't recognize that person sitting *there.* But in order to see a person there that she didn't recognize she had to hallucinate, and she had to hallucinate the circumstances of a previous time when I had used her as a subject and there was someone sitting there. So, she had to *regress* in order to *hallucinate* that person sitting there.

I did not ask her directly to regress. Instead, I talked about the last time I saw her, and where she was standing, and what did she remember, and she could state that she hadn't made any particular effort to remember the details I mentioned just now. And then I could put that question to her of whether or not she recognized that person sitting right *there,* and I certainly gave her the impression by the way I pointed that I meant that man, or that lady. I meant that person. And did she remember? Now, whenever you ask patients to do something, say it to them as if you absolutely expect them to do something about your question. Convey the clear message that your question is a legitimate one, a meaningful one, and that they are to cooperate.

"Is your right foot more numb than your left foot?" And you really want to know. You've asked a double bind question. There is no doubt in your voice that there is numbness of the feet. The patient has to examine that. The only doubt regards *which* foot is more numb, and the patient immediately re-established past learnings, past understandings, and develops that numbness.

Subtle Cues to Elict Hypnotic Phenomena

E: Now, take a deep breath and become wide awake. Let's see if I don't remember the date of that last meeting. Do you remember the date?

S: No, but there wasn't a table in the middle.

E: Who is the man sitting there?

S: I don't know.

154

E: You don't know. Thank you very much.

Now, of course, she corrected my memory, but she's gone back in the trance. Why should I be disturbed if I made a mistake? I shouldn't be concerned because it was a long time ago. She's at liberty to correct my mistake, my error. Why shouldn't she? And it does not interfere with the patient's capacity to respond.

Visual Hallucinations and Subtle Verbal Cues

[Erickson now addresses a woman named Marjorie.]

E: Marjorie, would you come over here? I noticed that you have been in a trance most of the time I have been talking. Why?

Marjorie (M): I just have to know.

E: You just have to know. All right, if you want certain learnings, certain understandings . . . tell me, Marjorie, do you think you will be able to forget anything that I tell you emphatically?

M: No, but . . .

E: Do you think you will be able to forget anything that I tell you emphatically?

M: I will never forget anything.

E: You will never forget anything. I told you some time ago that I do say the same things. [Erickson now tells a story that was lost in the recording.]

M: You have made me very happy.

E: I have made you very happy and you feel very puzzled.

155

You know, I think women should be both puzzling and puzzled.

M: Will I know sometime? [Apparently Marjorie has not yet found out what she wants to know.]

E: Certainly.

M: You won't have to be there?

E: That's right, why should I?

M: I just don't have to worry about it?

E: That's right. Now, do I have to tell you again, or clobber you over the head with my cane? [Laughter] By the way, where is Mary? Is that Mary over there? [Mary is Marjorie's daughter, whom Marjorie now proceeds to hallucinate.]

M: She ought to go to bed.

E: Why, is she in her pyjamas?

M: She's always in her pyjamas.

E: What color are her pyjamas?

M: Mauve, the same color I wear. You know Mary!

E: How is Mary?

M: She always laughs. When she laughs I have to laugh too, even if it isn't funny.

E: Even if it isn't funny, you laugh. How did you like that letter of inquiry I wrote Mary: "Mary, Mary, quite contrary, how does your ball point write?"

M: She doesn't show those kinds of letters to me anymore because I don't show her mine.

E: Where is Tommy? [Tommy is Marjorie's son.] Oh, there he is—no, *there* he is.

M: [I can't really see him.]

E: You don't think you will be able to see Tommy. Why not? You don't know? Why should you be bothered knowing? You see, I am interested in demonstrating certain things. By the way, do you know where you are?

M: Yes.

E: Where?

M: With you.*

E: With me, that's right—and with Mary.

M: She's gone now.

E: Just the two of us, all right. Now you really don't need to know why you can't see Tommy.

I am interested in the elicitation of certain psychological phenomena. I like to offer subjects suggestions and questions to see exactly how they handle things. To have a more effective demonstration, I might put intonations in my voice which negate the subject's performance; at other times, I might affirm the performance by another kind of intonation. The hypnotic subject responds to everything the operator puts out: to his words and ideas, to the implied meanings, to intonations and

---

Editors' Note: This is a very typical response of a subject in a deep trance: the psychological rapport with the hypnotherapist apparently overshadows or replaces all other forms of reality orientation.

inflections, to pauses, hesitations, uncertainties, to doubts, fears, and anxieties. Nothing is missed.

M: You like that, you really do.

E: I like what?

M: You like to feel Sandra around.

E: You know, Marjorie, you do have insight.

M: You enjoy this, like a fish in a bowl. You know it will work, I know it will work. I would like to know, but you are not going to tell me.

E: That is right, I am certainly not going to tell you why it will work out. You know it will work out, and I know it will work out, and that is sufficient. By the way, let's go to Los Angeles. Close your eyes and let's go to the Gourmet Restaurant. Now, take a deep breath and wake up. How did you get up here?

M: You must have asked me.

E: You wouldn't presume to walk up here all by yourself. I must have asked you—your subconscious knows that, right? Those are terrible pyjamas that Mary wears, aren't they?

M: They really are, they really are.

E: What can we do about a 14-year-old girl and her pyjamas?

M: Nothing.

E: You have learned that already? You didn't wait until she was 15. All girls are like that.

M: Even when they are 35!

E: Even when they are 35. By the way, where are we?

M: At the Gourmet Restaurant.

E: Do you recognize everybody?—they are all here.

I asked Marjorie, "Do you recognize everybody here?"; and she is still looking at me. She hasn't really come out of her trance. She is still in a trance, but a different type, a different level of hypnosis. She can talk with me, she can argue with me, she can dispute me; but I think you could do anything from major to minor surgery on Marjorie at this point. She can hallucinate at any level you are interested in hallucinating at, and yet she picked up that cue I gave her when I altered my voice about her son. You saw her ready hallucination of her daughter, Mary, followed by her failure to hallucinate her son, Tommy. To the inexperienced observer, it seemed that I asked Marjorie to hallucinate her son, but Marjorie didn't need much training to recognize my intonation and to understand it correctly.

Response Readiness: The Facility for Hypnotic Behavior

I first met Marjorie some time ago at the San Diego County Dental Society Meeting. I needed a subject. I looked over the audience while giving the general lecture, and when the time came for the demonstration I said, "I would like to have that lady over there."

Marjorie didn't believe that I meant her. It took some argument to convince her that I really did mean her, so she finally came up. Her first trance was like this one, and since there was no platform at that particular place, we had to stand up. So in the first hypnotic situation, Marjorie learned to go into a trance standing up. Why shouldn't she? It was perfectly easy, perfectly possible. The important thing is what is going on in the mind of the person you are working with.

PART III

EXPERIENTIAL LEARNINGS:
THE BASIS FOR HYPNOTIC BEHAVIOR*

What I want to discuss first is the nature of hypnotic trance and the nature of hypnotic induction. I want to give you a better understanding of what lies behind this kind of scientific work.

One of the first things I want to mention is this matter of learning. As we go through life we learn a great many things by experience. We learn things by experience we do not even know that we learn. A small child slaps a red-hot griddle just once and learns for the rest of his life not to slap a red-hot griddle.

To get a conditioned response in a psychology laboratory you have to set up stimulation for your laboratory student 50, 60, 100 times—and the student is much better educated than the infant! It takes a long time to teach that student to develop a conditioned response. Learning in life is one thing; learning in the laboratory or in the schoolroom is a totally different matter.

What are some of those experiential learnings that we acquire? A little baby looks at the pabulum and wonders, *What is that stuff?* The baby sees mother thinking—*Baby must eat the pabulum*—and the baby reads the mother's facial expression and knows that the pabulum does not taste good. Ever after that, the child can recognize that expression in the mother's face and respond in a similar way.

*Seminar given in Seattle, Washington, May 21-23, 1965, Section 1.

The little child has difficulty in locating his toes, his knees, his fingers. But eventually the child learns to recognize those various parts of the body so easily that when a mosquito lights on his right shoulder the child does not have to figure out: "Now, let's see—my left hand is here; I lift it up by bending the elbow, and then I move it medially, and then I can get it a little bit higher, and then I swat the mosquito." That mosquito would be well fed and long gone by the time the child got through that sort of analysis. The body senses the mosquito bite, and the rest of the body is conditioned to respond immediately to that particular stimulus: the child slaps the mosquito before stopping to analyze that it is on the right shoulder. That is what I mean by experiential learning. We have a tremendous number of such experiences. We learn by fear reaction to alter our blood content as Dr. Cheek just mentioned. We learn by smoking excessively to alter our patterns of behavior in many ways, and so on.

The Conscious and Unconscious Minds: Conflicts between Verbal and Nonverbal Behavior

In hypnosis one makes use of all these experiential learnings in order to direct and organize the patient's behavior. All of you know the conscious mind; all of you know the unconscious mind. They are separate and distinct. The unconscious mind goes with you wherever you go, but your unconscious thinking is not necessarily known to your conscious mind. You can think one thing consciously while your unconscious mind thinks the exact opposite. When Dr. Cheek mentioned certain ideas in this area I recalled a patient of mine who really illustrated this point. That patient said to me, "When I was first married I wanted to have a lot of children." I heard his words and I understood his words, but I also understood the shaking of his head in a negative fashion. That is why I have found it extremely informative to let patients verbalize while I notice their *physical* behavior—which often disputes what they are verbalizing.

Hypnotic Induction via Inward Focusing: Revival of Past Experiential Learnings

What does one do in hypnosis to produce a trance? It certainly is not a matter of having an eagle eye, or being six feet tall, or anything of that sort. The hypnosis that develops in any situation is the hypnosis that develops within the patient. *The patient does his own development of the hypnotic trance.* He does it by listening to you, and if you are sufficiently interesting, if you can secure his attention and secure his cooperation, the patient is then going to limit and restrict his behavior to you and to what you are saying; the patient is going to understand what you have said; the patient is going to be willing to receive what you have said uncritically—and when I say uncritically I am speaking in the scientific sense of the word. Most of us do not accept things uncritically. If I were to ask any one of you to take off your coat, your immediate reply would be, "Why?" It would be a critical response. But if I asked you as a hypnotic subject to take off your coat, your thinking might be: "Now that is something I can do. It is perfectly possible. It is suitable in this situation. Now, is there a need?" Certainly the doctor wouldn't ask the patient to do it if there were not a need, and therefore the patient would make the decision after having examined the idea and examined it thoroughly for its intrinsic values. Then he would decide whether or not to execute the request.

In inducing a trance you ask your patient to give you his full attention. You don't want him counting the spots on the wall; you don't want him tinkering with his watch and shaking it to see if it is still running. You want him to give you his full attention and to give it to you so intently that he is not going to notice anything else. And as he attends to you he is cutting down his field of visual awareness; he is cutting down his field of auditory awareness; and he is directing his thinking and his feeling to within himself. At that point you can suggest to the patient that as he looks at any spot he wishes, or looks off into the distance, he can feel himself relaxing. You are not really relaxing that patient. *You are asking him to revive his memories and his understandings of what physical relaxation is.* And as he begins to revive those memories and understandings, his body begins to relax and to experience that relaxation, and he finds it the same as those experiential learnings that brought about relaxation for him in the past. As he relaxes more and more you can suggest that his legs and arms can feel heavy and tired and comfortable. What are you doing? You are simply asking the patient to review his memories and his understandings of heaviness, of tiredness, of comfort; and as he directs his attention more and more to within himself you are setting the foundation for him to draw upon any experiential learnings that he has had in his life.

If I were to ask any one of you to raise your blood pressure 20 points at my request, you would immediately doubt your ability to do so. In medical school I discovered, both as a student and later as a teacher, that medical students could do this kind of thing quite easily. They could alter blood circulation in specific areas of their bodies, or they could alter smooth muscle functioning. All you needed to do was announce, "There will be a written quiz today," and they would divide into the reading group and the smooth muscle group, and they would do it so quickly and so easily!* It's all a matter of experiential learnings, experiential learnings of the body. When Dr. Cheek wants a patient to feel comfortable in regard to bleeding, why shouldn't he use the same technique that he used in medical school when the unexpected written quizzes were ordered?

Hypnotic Induction: Many Appraoches to Inner Focusing

There are many different techniques that one can use to induce hypnotic trance. One of them is the eye fixation relaxa-

---

Editors' Note: This transcription does not make sense. Erickson apparently is trying to make the point that in any group situation, some people will experience their emotionality by exaggerated parasympathetic responses and others by disturbances in the sympathetic system.

tion technique; another is simply a matter of closing the eyes and going deeper and deeper asleep. I mention these techniques because *all hypnotic techniques are centered primarily around directing the patient's attention to within himself.* The verbalizations you use—whether you suggest that the patient's hand levitate higher and higher and higher, or whether you suggest he relax more and more, or whether you suggest that his eyes close bit by bit until they are fully closed—are really all for your own education. Using different approaches gives you the opportunity to learn how to talk to patients and to learn how to direct their attention within themselves. I don't think it makes any difference what kind of a technique you use. The technique is verbal on your part, but your technique centers entirely around the patient's own responses.

The Permissive Technique: Engaging the Patient's Cooperation and Evoking Unconscious Potentials

Now I would like to dicuss the matter of producing results. When you want to ask your patient to do something, I think it is a very serious error not to ask him first to cooperate with you—unless, of course, you have a specific reason for not doing so. I like to use a permissive technique. In certain cases, however, you may need to use an authoritative technique: "I WANT YOU TO MOVE YOUR FINGER." When a patient rouses from trance in the middle of his operation the anesthesiologist can say very sweetly but very emphatically: "Now that you have awakened and you notice that everything is fine, you might as well go right back to sleep."* And the anesthesiologist ought to mean that and to say it in a sufficiently authoritative fashion so that the patient responds. But to elicit the cooperation of the patient one ought to be permissive for best results. One really

Editors' Note: This is an unusually clear example of a compound suggestion where a labeling of the patient's ongoing behavior in the first phrase, "Now that you have awakened," is an undeniable truth that tends to structure a yes set for the acceptance of the suggestions that immediately follow: "everything is fine," and "go right back to sleep." See *Hypnotherapy.*

ought to ask the patient to cooperate in achieving a common goal. You should keep in mind that that common goal is a goal for the welfare of the patient wherein the patient is cooperating with you to achieve something that primarily is of benefit to him. He cooperates with the surgeon primarily to get over whatever the condition is.

The average patient has little conception of what he can do— [of what his potentials are]. I mentioned raising the blood pressure a few minutes ago. I know just one word you need utter to a Democrat during an election in order to raise his blood pressure, and there are many other similar situations. But just as you can raise the blood pressure, so also can you drop it; and I think you ought to bear that in mind when you are dealing with a patient. You say something terribly threatening to a patient and his heart drops down to the bottom of his shoes. He just falls down completely. He collapses, and yet he is sitting right there and he is not the least bit collapsed. But I am speaking of an inner response, and as you listen to that defeat I think you should have had in mind, if not consciously at least unconsciously, some of your own unconscious learnings in this matter of altering responses.

You ought to attempt to elicit responses in a permissive fashion. You can do this by educating the patient in regard to his own potentials. We all can do so many more things than we realize. You can ask a hypnotic subject to develop, let us say, hypnotic deafness, and he will respond: "I can't develop deafness!" Yet we do develop deafness as a matter of course in our everyday lives. We become unaware of certain sounds. The air conditioning is not noticed until it suddenly goes off. You can be reading a paper or a book and your wife speaks to you. Ten minutes later she asks, "Aren't you going to answer?", and you respond, "Answer what?" How do you develop that deafness?

One uses hypnosis by directing the patient's attention inward, and then asking him to utilize all the potentials of his experiential learnings. That utilization can involve all manner of physiological processes, psychological responses, and any neurological functionings.

166

Utilizing Resistance

Sometimes resistive patients want to establish contests with you; sometimes they are simply afraid of you. It is up to you to diagnose which is the case. Is this to be a contest? Or is this patient afraid? If it is a contest you might as well quit right then and there, because you are going to lose that contest. *Your task is to transform the situation into one which is not a contest.* And if the patient is afraid it is up to you to discuss the matter.

I will give you an example of a resistant patient who wanted a contest. She came into my office and announced: "Dr. Cheek has tried to hypnotize me without success. Several of his friends have also tried and failed. So I have come all the way from San Francisco to Phoenix so that you can fail too!"

My response was: "Well, I concede failure right now. But you do smoke four packages of cigarettes a day; you do have emphysema; you are worried about your heart. I think we ought to take up a discussion of that, and since you are intending to let me fail to hypnotize you, let me help you out. Just look at that clock on my desk right there. It is an ordinary clock. It is a green stamp clock, and you just look at it and keep your eyes wide open and stay fully awake—completely, fully awake—and just listen to what I have to say to you about emphysema and smoking and about your fears of your cardiac condition."

She kept her eyes on the clock and she listened. She listened so completely that at the end of two hours she didn't know that two hours had elapsed. She thought she had just sat down in the office. All I did was circumvent her resistance by asking her to limit her gaze entirely to that clock. She couldn't see the filing cabinet, the bookcases, the pictures on the wall, my desk, or anything else. Her attention was directed entirely within herself, completely within herself, and she was taken up with the question of whether she should quit smoking. Should she quit smoking? Should she quit smoking because she was afraid of dying of heart disease? Should she quit smoking because she was afraid of emphysema? What should she do about that? How could she learn to quit smoking?

She was one type of resistant patient where I just walked around the contest. One always wants to use whatever a resistant patient brings into the office. If you are going to practice medicine on a patient with an ulcer you had better make use of that ulcer in some way. If it is an appendix you had better use that appendix in some way. If the patient is as resistive as can be, you'd better use that resistance in some way.

The Indirect Hypnotic Development of Anesthesia for the Control of Pain

[Erickson now answers a question from the audience that was lost in the recording.] Pertinent to your question is a puzzle that has confronted me on a number of occasions. I have treated patients who were suffering from very severe terminal illnesses such as cancer and were obviously in a great deal of pain. Everything about them indicated they were suffering pain, including their neurological examinations. What I discovered was that I could put them in a trance and have them lose their pain without suggesting an anesthesia or an analgesia. Whether that happened because they equated going into a trance with being anesthetized, I really don't know. I told patients, "I am going to teach you first how to go into a hypnotic trance, and then, after you have learned that thoroughly, I will teach you about controlling the pain." Maybe these patients found a shortcut to their own learnings.

Utilizing Resistance in the Control of Pain: Cathy's Horrible Chanting

I am not going to give you a formal address tonight. Instead, I am going to present instances in which hypnosis was used successfully. One of the first instances I want to present concerned a 36-year-old woman dying of cancer who had three sons, ages 11, 9, and 7. Cathy was referred to me as a patient, and the doctor who referred her gave me the following information: "My patient has had everything possible in the way of surgery, everything possible in the way of X-ray therapy and implantations, and every kind of narcotic. Now nothing stops her pain. Would you try using hypnosis on her to give her some relief in the short time she has left?"

I made a house call on this patient. Upon entering the living-room I heard a rather horrible chanting coming from the bed-room: "Don't hurt me, don't hurt me, don't hurt me; don't scare me, don't scare me, don't hurt me; don't scare me, don't scare me, don't hurt me!"

Inquiry disclosed that Cathy was crying out these pleas every waking moment. It was utterly hideous to listen to her. I asked myself what sort of hypnotic technique could appease a patient who is behaving in such a manner?

Participating in Patient Behavior to Secure and Fixate Attention

I entered the bedroom and observed that Cathy was lying on her right side, all curled up, eyes closed, and chanting away. I listened to her for twenty to thirty minutes, trying to pick up the emphasis and rhythm of what she was saying. After I had listened for what I thought was enough time to learn all that, I began chanting with her: "I am going to hurt you, I am going to hurt you, I am going to hurt you, I am going to hurt you; I am going to scare you, I am going to scare you, I am going to hurt you."

I kept time with her, and after about ten minutes of that joint chanting Cathy opened her eyes, looked at me, and said, "Why do you want to hurt me?" I replied, "I want to help you, too." She resumed her chant and I resumed mine.

A few minutes later Cathy asked, "How are you going to hurt me?" I answered, "By teaching you something that you need to know." She resumed chanting, and I joined in.

Another few minutes passed and she again asked me questions about what I planned to do; she wanted to know just how I was going to hurt her.

"It is very simple," I explained. You are lying on your right side all curled up, so I am going to have you turn over in bed, but don't move your body—just *mentally* turn over in bed. Think it through. Think out how you move your arms, how you move your shoulders, how you move your legs, how you move your body, and when you are all turned over mentally, tell me so."

Cathy kept breaking into chants and I kept joining her, and that would bring her back to the task of turning over in bed.

Finally she announced, "I am all turned over."

"All right," I replied. "Now I am going to hurt you some more. I am going to ask you to turn to the other side." She turned to the other side mentally.

Then she asked, "Now why did you do that?"

"I want to teach you something," I answered. "I wanted to teach you that I could hurt you, but if I can hurt you, it ought to be reasonable that I can also *stop* hurting you; and if *I* can stop hurting you, I can gradually stop *you* from hurting you."

That seemed to interest her a great deal, and so I pointed out to her that the doctor had told me some bad things about her.

"Yes," she agreed, "I am going to die inside of ten months, and I don't want to die, and I have a lot of pain. They can't do anything with it. They can't give me medicine. They can't do anything for me."

"That is why I am here," I told her, "to do something about it. And I started by scaring you and by hurting you, and now you know, and you know very definitely, that I can do things *to* you and *for* you."

Now that may have been too sophisticated an argument, but it did teach her that I could do something to, and perhaps for, her.*

Next I questioned her about her malignancy. She had had her right breast removed, but the cancer had nonetheless metastasized throughout her entire body—into the hip bones and into the spine, so that she had pain throughout her legs as well.

Editors' Note: Precisely because it was a "sophisticated" argument—that is, new and unusual for her—it absorbed and focused her attention in a hypnotic manner, thereby evoking latent potentials that are usually suppressed in our typical, everyday reality orientation. See "Psychological Shocks and Creative Movements," in Vol. IV of *Collected Papers.*

Confusion to Evoke Receptivity and Facilitate Indirect Analegisa

I told her that the next bit of teaching I was going to give her was something that she just wouldn't understand, but that I wanted her to listen to me until she could actually do the thing I told her to do. I told her she was to develop one of the most awful, most terrible, and most unbearable itches she had ever had in her life on the sole of her right foot.

"Why would I do that?" she asked.

"Because," I said, "I am the doctor here and you are the patient. You go ahead and develop that itch."

She tried very, very hard to develop the itch, and finally she apologized by stating that the best she could do was to get a numb feeling in the back of her right foot. I settled for that numbness right then and there.

[How did this happen?] When she attempted to develop that itch without understanding the purpose or meaning of what I was driving at, her very confusion and lack of understanding rendered her willing to open her mind to any understanding that I might give her. So I settled for that numbness as soon as she developed it.

"Cathy," I said, "I want you to study that numbness because something is going to happen to it. It is going to spread up over your ankle, up the front of your leg, up the calf of your leg, clear up to the knee. It is going to go past your knee, it is going to go way up to your hips, and way up to the middle part of your abdomen, and then it is going to cross over and travel down your left leg clear to the sole of the left foot."

In that nice trance Cathy proceeded to get the left leg as numb as the right leg.

She already felt very relieved and very grateful for the loss of her pain, but the question of what to do next then arose.

"Cathy," I proceeded, "now we will start the numbness going up either the right side of your body or the left side of your body. We started with your right foot. Maybe it would be only fair to start with the left side of your body."

I wanted to work with the left side of her body because her malignancy had been in the right breast, and therefore I

171

had better keep over on the left side of her body. So I produced a numbness slowly, letting it creep up higher and higher until it reached her shoulder. Then the numbness crossed over to her right shoulder and moved upward from her waistline until it covered all of the right side of her chest except one area. And I explained to her with profound apologies that even though I had relieved the pain of her cancer by this numbness I would have to confess that I was going to be an absolute failure in one regard. I would not be able to remove the pain from the site of the surgical scar. Instead of removing absolutely all of the pain, the best, the very best, that I could do would be to leave the scar area with an annoying, disagreeable, great-big-mosquito-like feeling. It would be something awfully annoying; something she would feel helpless about; something she would wish would stop. But *it would be endurable,* and I impressed that point on Cathy's mind. It took me four hours to accomplish everything.

I had visited Cathy for the first time on February 26th. I saw her a couple of weeks later, in March, for about an hour. I saw her the latter part of March for about an hour, and I saw her for about twenty minutes in April.

In one session, I told Cathy that she really ought to eat more, and I spent quite a bit of time with her explaining how good beef steak tasted and suggesting that she eat more of it because she had been losing weight too rapidly. She developed a good appetite, and by the time I left she was having her companion cook a steak for her.

I didn't see Cathy again until July, and it was obvious to me that she didn't have much longer to live. She was still free of pain except for that mosquito-bite feeling at the site of the operation. Then, in the first week of August, Cathy was conversing with a friend when she suddenly became unconscious and died two hours later.

Now let's analyze what I did in this case. I had to get in touch with Cathy. Cathy was presenting a terrible barrier to me. The only way I could possibly approach her was to join with her and that joining would compel her to notice me. She was employing that chanting to take her mind off her pain, and she

172

couldn't share that pain with anybody; yet I forceably made her share it with me. People do sing, hum, or groan; they will keep up a dirge of some sort to take their minds off pain, and Cathy was doing precisely that. So I simply joined in. It wasn't my chant; it was hers. And that allowed her to question me irritably about what I meant by chanting, "I am going to hurt you, I am going to scare you."

Next, I wanted to impress on Cathy that I could do things with her. For me to have marched in and said, "I can lessen your cancer pain," would have been an utterly stupid thing to do. All the other doctors had failed to lessen her pain, and she knew it. They had given her a prognosis of two months, and for me to have walked in, a total stranger, and announced, "I am going to hypnotize you out of your pain," would have been simply assinine. Instead, I showed her that I could hurt her, and that was entirely reasonable. She wouldn't want it done; she would feel helpless about it; and so I proceeded to hurt her. I was demonstrating that she was helpless in my hands, that I could do things to her.

Realistic Pain Removal: Leaving an Itch to Reinforce the Absence of Pain

Then I suggested an itch on the sole of her foot—as far away from the site of the operation as possible. And, of course, she failed by producing a numbness instead. Now, what did that patient really want—an itch, or a numbness? It was she who produced the numbness, and I simply was intelligent enough to use that numbness and to spread it over her body; over the legs first, again keeping away from the cancer site, and then moving it upward toward her chest.

I did not make the mistake that many doctors make of being too purposed and too encompassing in what they try to accomplish with a patient. Cathy had pain, and Cathy knew that she was going to die, and I had better leave her with a little endurable pain. For the remainder of her life— from February 26th to the day of her death in August—Cathy could wonder why I hadn't been able to take away that little bit of an itch *when I had been able to take away all that severe pain.* That is what I wanted Cathy to think. I wanted her to reinforce the fact that *all the serious pain was gone,* and that it was just lamentable that that little bit of an annoying itch remained.

Fixating Attention to Induce Unexpected Trance

I will give you another case example, and perhaps this will also answer Dr. F's question about why I have never been arrested. [Laughter]

I was in an airport in Denver, Colorado, at two o'clock in the morning waiting for my plane. I saw a tired mother coming into the waiting area with five children, all of whom were dragging their feet, whining, and whimpering. You know how children can really cut up at two o'clock in the morning when they would rather be in bed.

These children were really raising a row with their mother, and she was saying so patiently, "Now, Johnnie, sit here, please; Mary, sit there, please."

I watched that scene for awhile. Then I went and got a big newspaper and returned. I stood in front of those kids and slowly tore a tiny strip the whole length of the paper and laid it down on the floor. I rapidly gained an attentive audience of six.

I tore another strip and I laid it crosswise. I tore another, and then I tore another, and I made quite a pattern on the floor. Then I went over and sat on the bench beside the oldest child, and I tore little, short strips and laid them in a pattern on the seat beside the child.

"This is what I always do before I go to sleep," I told him. "When you look at those strips, you will also get sleepy."

I took hold of his hand, lifted it up producing a catalepsy, and then laid his arm very gently on his leg, dropping my hand down in front of his eyes. His eyes closed and I turned to the next child.

The mother was watching me with a great deal of interest and when I finally finished with all five children, she looked up, saw her husband coming, and said to him: "Oh, John, Dr. Erickson has just hypnotized the kids for me."

I met her at a seminar a few years later, and she asked, "Do you still go around hypnotizing little children with newspapers?"

The Double Bind: Illusory Choice to Cover All Possibilities except Failure: Joe's Dry Bed

Another example I want to cite illustrates [a linguistic tool] that is very important in facilitating hypnosis: namely, the use of the double bind. By the double bind I mean making a statement in such a way that the person thinks he has a choice when he really does not have a choice. For example, I have never asked my children to go to bed at eight o'clock. Instead I would ask them, "Do you want to go to bed at eight o'clock, or at a quarter before eight? It was they who would say, "At eight o'clock!" I didn't need to say it. And at the dinner table, I would ask, "Do you want a large helping of this vegetable, or just a medium helping?", when the expression on their faces said, "None at all!"

A twelve-year-old boy was brought to me by his parents. He had not had a dry bed for twelve years. He had been spanked, he had been thoroughly stitched; he had been deprived of his meals, he had been deprived of water; he had been cystoscoped, I don't know how many times; and he had had countless barrels of atropine sulphate, and of all the other things that doctors give to torture enuretics. The father and the mother explained how they had rubbed his face in the wet bed, how they had spanked him, how they had inflicted every possible indignity upon him.

I began by telling the parents who would do what: "All right, you have explained the case to me. Your son is twelve years old. He is my patient now, and I think it is only ethical that you keep your cotton-picking paws off my patient. Don't mention wet bed, don't mention dry bed, don't even say the word *bed* in his presence. He is my patient and I am handling this!" I put it across to the parents that they were to keep well out of my range.

I called Joe into the office. "This is the second day of January," I explained, "and you have wet the bed, your parents say, every night for twelve years. You know that and I know that, so now let us forget about it. Let us talk about something that is really important.

"Now, this is the second of January, and I don't think it would be reasonable, not the least bit reasonable in any way, for me to expect you to have a permanently dry bed two weeks from now. And you know, by that time January will be practically over, and then February is a short month. Does anybody want to dispute that? It is a short month, and I certainly don't think you ought to start a permanently dry bed before March. It doesn't seem reasonable that you do it before then, but I will tell you what you might be interested in doing.

"In a couple of weeks from now (I pointed to the calendar on the wall), I would like to have you puzzle mentally over this question: *In two weeks from today, will it be on Wednesday, or will it be on Thursday, that I will have a dry bed for the first time?* Two weeks from now. *Will it be on Wednesday, or will it be on Thursday, that I will have my first dry bed?* And you will have to wait until Friday morning to know for certain, and so that Friday you will come in to tell me whether it was Wednesday or whether it was Thursday."

Joe came in that Friday morning and said, "You know, it was both nights!"

Now what had I done? I had put him in a double bind. He had to expect one of those two nights for his first dry bed. He didn't really know which night he would be dry, and he surprised himself.

"February is such a short month," I continued, "that you really ought not to have a dry bed, reasonably speaking, more than three times in any one of those four weeks of February— three times in succession in any one of those weeks. Now that doesn't mean you can't have one dry bed or two dry beds, but I don't think it would be reasonable to expect more than three dry beds in any one of those four weeks."

Joe's bed began drying up with great rapidity, and at the end of February I said: "Now, I still don't know when your permanently dry bed will come about, but you are Irish and St. Patrick's Day is a very nice day; but when I think about how your father and mother have treated you, I think April Fools also would be a very nice day. There is one thing I would like you to get straight, Joe, and that is that when you have your dry bed, whether it is on St. Patrick's Day or April Fools Day or any day in between, *that day is your business.* It is none of my business. It is nobody else's business either."

I don't know when Joe began his permanently dry bed, but Joe is now a dentist. He uses hypnosis. He has had a permanently dry bed since somewhere between St. Patrick's Day and April Fools Day of his twelfth year, and it is none of my business. Joe has been in the office many times since then to discuss various issues. The day of his permanently dry bed is still a secret, and he still laughs about it because it isn't my business.

Let the child pick his own time for having a permanently dry bed. Let the child pick his own time in his own way. The fact that you set it up in the form of a double bind doesn't alter the therapeutic situation at all. I think it is awfully important to use double binds to make certain that your patient is going to respond adequately.

"Talking Sense" to Divert Attention and Control Pain: Robert's Red Blood and Ten Stitches

Several years ago my three-year-old son, Robert, fell down the back steps and drove a tooth up into the maxilla. Now being just three years old he was quite frightened and suffering a great deal of pain. He lay on his back on the pavement, crying to high heaven his expectations for a lifetime of agony in blood.

His mother and I ran out to the backyard to see what all the hullabaloo was about. As I looked down at Robert screaming and crying, I knew one thing that he did not know: I knew that there is a right time to speak to a child and that time is when the child is able to listen to you. While Robert was screaming he would not be listening to me, but I knew his wind would run out and that he would have to take a deep breath to recharge his battery. So when he paused to take that breath, I said, "And it hurts just terribly, doesn't it Robert?"

Now at that point he knew I was talking sense. Most parents

177

do not talk sense to their children. Robert went on with the screaming and took another breath, and I said, "And it will keep right on hurting." That was exactly what Robert was worrying about. He was afraid it would keep right on hurting, so again I had spoken intelligently.

Then when he paused for breath the third time I said, "Maybe the pain will go away in a minute or two." What three-year-old hasn't heard the phrase, *a minute or two?* That was old stuff to Robert, but it did give him a faint ray of hope.

When Robert paused for the next breath I signaled his mother and we both looked at the blood stains on the pavement, and I said, "Mother, is that good, red, strong blood?" She looked as worried as I did. We both looked at the blood, and Robert's eyes bugged out as he looked at it. Mother and I debated the issue of the quality of Robert's blood, and then I reasoned:

"You know, Robert, the color of the pavement makes it difficult to see if your blood is the best kind of good, red, strong blood. You've got to see the blood where it is nice and white."

So Mrs. Erickson and I picked up Robert and took him to the bathroom and let his blood dribble into the nice, white sink. And you know, it was good, red, strong blood, and Robert was just as interested as I was.

Next I wondered, Would Robert's blood mix well with water and make the right color of pink? I washed Robert's face and it did make the right color pink.

Then I broke the really bad news to Robert. "You can count to ten easily," I reasoned. "You can count to twenty easily, but, you know, when the doctor puts the stitches in your lip I don't think he could put in twenty stitches that you could count. I don't think he could even put in ten. But you go ahead and count the stitches and see if he can put in at least ten."

So Robert went off to the doctor's with a wonderful goal in mind: he was going to count those stitches!

When we arrived at the doctor's office the surgeon said, "I don't want to inject a local and I don't want to give him a general."

"Just go ahead and sew it up," Mrs. Erickson directed.

And so he did begin to sew up Robert's injury, and Robert dutifully began to count: "One . . . two . . . three . . ."

In the end, Robert got only seven stitches, and all the while the surgeon kept looking from Robert to Mrs. Erickson and back to Robert. [He just didn't understand a three-year-old child wanting *more* stitches!]

Pupil Dilation via Imagination: Betty Alice's Practical Joke

Everyone in my family likes to play practical jokes. [My daughter, Betty Alice, once played a practical joke on a doctor that very nicely illustrated how the mind can affect the body.] When she was ten years old, we discovered that Betty Alice had a strabismus and needed glasses. She went to the opthamologist to get her vision corrected, and she had to wear a patch for awhile. Now Betty Alice was a curious little girl. She had to do some exercises with her eyes, and she would sit in front of a mirror and very carefully practice those exercises.

One day she went to the opthamologist for a check-up. He sat her down and proceeded to examine her right eye in a very thorough way by measuring the diameter of the pupil, and so on. Then he read over all his notations, shifted his examination to the left eye, and almost fell off his seat. The right pupil was of normal size, but the left pupil was very widely dilated. He looked alarmed. He checked that right eye very carefully, and then he examined the left eye with the widely dilated pupil. He put it all down in his notations, re-read them, and then looked back at her right eye. Now the right eye was widely dilated and the left eye was contracted, so he began to *re*-examine the right eye!

Suddenly Betty Alice burst out into giggles, saying, "I did that on purpose!"

"How?" asked a very disconcerted opthamologist.

"You learn to look with one eye when you wear a patch," Betty Alice explained. "Then you can *imagine* that there is a patch in front of your eye when there really isn't; and then you look way, way off into the distance, or you look up and you imagine you see clouds, and then you imagine you are seeing with the other eye and you do the same thing, and if you do that often enough soon you can dilate your pupil whenever you want to—the right one, the left one, or both of them!"

"Let me see you do it," the doctor said.

Betty Alice promptly proceeded to dilate the right and then the left; to dilate the left and to contract the right, and so on. The doctor became quite convinced of what kids can do!

The Power of Mental Mechanisms: Self-Induced Death

Here is another example which [shows the mental mechanisms that carry out hypnotic suggestion].

During my psychiatric internship at the Colorado Psychiatric Hospital a patient came in one day and announced, "I am going to die next Saturday morning." The Chief-of-Staff said to us, "Here is a man we will keep under observation twenty-four hours a day." We had the man examined in every conceivable way; gave him every physiological test and every psychological test, and all the patient would say was, "I am dying on Saturday. I am dying on Saturday, at ten o'clock in the morning, on such-and-such a date."

The man slept well and he ate well. His blood pressure was fine, his blood chemistry was fine, every index from his physical examination was fine. Saturday morning we all gathered around and watched that patient die at ten o'clock. The autopsy showed no reason whatsoever for the patient's death.

Many studies in the literature on psychosomatic medicine report this peculiar kind of death. You see the same phenomenon in primitive peoples, when they say they are going to die as a result of a hexing or voodoo of some sort. Self-induced death is tremendously interesting because it shows the effects of thoughts and feelings and attitudes and beliefs on the functioning of the human body. You can observe the most surprising things that happen to people as a result of their beliefs and their feelings. [These same mechanisms are the ones you try to direct and utilize in a positive way in hypnosis.]

Psychosomatic Medicine: Precursor for Modern Medical Applications of Hypnosis

Hypnosis has long been recognized by people, but its history in terms of scientific recognition has been rather short. This is because hypnosis has been regarded as a matter of mysticism, cultism, and superstition. [But hypnosis is really a matter of mental mechanisms,] and why shouldn't science be interested in the functioning of those mechanisms? The brain cells do control the body in a great variety of ways—neurologically, physiologically, and psychologically as well.

Hypnosis really got its start in modern medicine in the second decade of this century when people became interested in that peculiar concept called "psychosomatic medicine." Frances Dunbar was very much criticized and ostracized when she first began her studies on psychosomatic medicine, because who on earth was going to believe that business worries, or marital worries, or any kind of worries in the head could result in ulcers of the stomach!

Yet, the general public adopted that notion, understanding that worries, be they real or imaginary, could produce a great many physical complaints and physiological alterations. And because the general public got behind the notion of psychosomatic medicine, the physicians who were so dubious about it were literally forced to consider and investigate it. With this recognition of the importance of brain/mind functioning on the rest of the body and the subsequent development of psychosomatic medicine, provision was made at last for the introduction of hypnosis as an adjunctive technique in the practice of medicine.

Brain Functioning: Vast Capacities for New and Lost Learnings: Lashley's Experiments

We really don't know how the brain functions. There are too many billions of brain cells for us to have a very accurate concept of the complexity of brain alterations. And when you look at body chemistry you see the same complexity: how only a small amount of any particular substance is required to produce phenomenal changes in the body. It was mentioned this morning that 1/500,000 of a milligram of secretin would activate the gallbladder. Now that isn't a very large amount, but it can produce a tremendous reaction in the gallbladder which affects all digestive processes. So how much does the functioning of one brain cell, or of patterns of brain cells, alter the functioning of the human body?

The rat experiments conducted by Lashley in the 1920s come to mind. First, Lashley taught rats to run a maze. Then he operated on the brains of those rats to discover where the information on running the maze was stored and proceeded to destroy those original learning pathways. Now he put the rats back in the maze and had them learn to run it for a second time. A great deal of experimental surgery was necessary to discover where the second learning pathways had formed. Lashley repeated the whole cycle, destroying the second learning pathway, and having the rats learn yet another time. I think, all together, Lashley taught those same rats how to run the maze by using five different brain pathways. Temple Bailey did the same thing, and the experiment has since been repeated by many investigators. What it demonstrates is that *when one part of the brain is damaged you can call upon another part of the brain to develop the lost learning.*

Hypnosis and Brain Functioning: New Ideas to Evoke Untapped Potentials: Amnesia and Pain Control

In hypnosis we offer ideas to a patient, to a person, to a subject. We ask the individual to learn out of his wealth of brain cells—out of his wealth of potential capacities—some new and different way to function. When the individual can be truly uncritical—when he is willing to receive an idea for the purpose of examining it—only then can hypnosis be effective. *Hypnosis is a means of communicating ideas; it is a means of asking people to accept ideas for examination, to discover the intrinsic meanings, and then to decide whether or not to act upon those particular meanings.*

What are the behaviors you can perform under hypnosis? There really is no behavior you can carry out in the hypnotized state that you cannot carry out in the ordinary, everyday waking state. The advantage with hypnosis is that you can control, direct, and prolong that behavior that just pops up in ordinary, everyday life. Perhaps the best example is amnesia. If I were to ask any one of you to forget some specific item, you would have very great difficulty doing so in your ordinary, waking state. But how many times have you been introduced to a person, been told the person's name, repeated the name, shook hands with the full resolution of remembering that name you have been told; and yet the moment you drop the hand you forget the name? Instant forgetting is as easy in the ordinary waking state, despite your wishes, as it is in the hypnotic state. And so you make use of hypnosis to ask people to function as they do in ordinary, everyday life but to do so at a given time, and for a given length of time. You ask them to use experiential learnings and capacities in ways of which they were formerly unaware.

Most of us don't really know what we are capable of doing. You think you cannot control pain, and yet every dentist can tell you how easily patients lose their toothaches on the way to the dental office. Every one of you knows that you can have a splitting headache and lose it while watching a suspenseful movie; you lose it *not* because you have received an intravenous injection for pain, but because your attention has been drawn to more compelling matters—even though that headache was the most compelling matter a few minutes ago.

You have very severe pain, drastic pain, and yet, let something happen that takes your attention away from that pain and you will lose it. The most compelling worries, fears, anxieties, and pains can be lost instantaneously at the sight of an automobile accident. You simply forget them. How does the brain manage to abolish overwhelming subjective experiences just because another visual experience intervenes? In hypnosis you are calling upon that vast array of brain cells with which we are all endowed but of which we are virtually unaware.

The point I want to stress in these introductory remarks is that we actually know very, very little about brain functioning, about human physiology, about human neurology; and that we ought to remain completely openminded about all the possibilities for combining and permuting those countless, billions of brain cells.

Associating Trance with Behavioral Inevitabilities via the Negative; Contingent Suggestions for Awakening

I would like to demonstrate a technique I use very frequently. It is not usually a time-consuming technique, but today I am going to slow it down for the purpose of demonstration. I am going to ask someone to volunteer—someone who has not been a hypnotic subject before. [Apparently, a person from the audience rises and begins to come forward. Erickson begins a trance induction.]

E: Now there is no hurry at all about coming forward. When you get to the aisle, just stop and wait. Now, what I would like to have you do is this: Walk up here very, very slowly, and in walking slowly, I would like you to be very sure that *you do not go into a trance state until you sit down here in this chair.* Now come forward very slowly, with your hands by your side, slower, slower. That's it, and make up your mind *not to go into a trance until you sit down in this chair.* Now stand in front of it, and slowly get ready, and slowly sit down, and close your eyes, and take a deep breath, and go deeper and deeper into a trance.

And when you begin to realize that you are going deeper and deeper—when you begin to realize that, and not until you begin to realize that you are going deeper and deeper—you will notice that your head is slowly lowering toward your chest, and a bit more, and your head will slowly lower a bit more, very slowly as you realize it more and more. And then as you realize that you are about to awaken, your left hand will slowly begin to lower toward your lap, and when it reaches your lap, you will be wide awake, alert, feeling refreshed. What would you like to say?

S: Nothing in particular.

E: Nothing in particular to say.

S: I really don't know.

E: Did you know that you were lowering your head? You suddenly altered the movements of your body completely. You were all set when you got right there, where the floor tends to level off. You roused a bit when you touched the railing with your hand. You came over here and I made you hesitate; I made you hesitate so that you would have a chance to reestablish the feeling you had when you reached the level part of the floor. And then when you sat down what happened? I had you close your eyes. What else? After a while I lifted your arm up.

Notice the ironing out of the facial expression that occurs immediately, as well as the lack of attention to what I am saying to the audience. If I were to speak about any one of you, you would immediately become self-conscious, yet our volunteer here shows very little self-consciousness, and she shows no tendency to turn her head toward me even though I am speaking about her. There is also a difference in the way she holds her hand up.

I have said to many patients as they entered my office, "Please do not go into a trance until you have seated yourself comfortably in the chair." [What is really in this simple request?] There are two separate tasks here: the first is to sit down in the chair, and the second is to become comfortable. Patients do not realize that there are two separate tasks in the request. And what happens when they carry out those two tasks?

185

Now I know that when patients enter the office they are going to sit down in a chair, and I also know that they want to be comfortable in that chair. I merely tie this matter of going into a hypnotic trance into a task that I know they are going to carry out automatically; and since they are going to sit down in the chair, and since they do want to be comfortable, I merely add to those two tasks a simple third task: namely, to go into a trance after they sit down in the chair. Only I phrase the request negatively because then there is no reason for patients to resist [since the resistance is indirectly discharged by my use of the negative]; so the request satisfies patients, and it meets the situation very adequately.

Hypnosis as Inner Absorption and Self-Examination

[Now there is verbal interaction between Erickson and the audience which was lost in the recording. At the point when the tape resumes, an audience member is apparently clarifying something Erickson has just said.]

Q: You mean not mention the word *hypnosis?* You never do use it, do you?

E: Not very often. You have trouble with your wife and she has trouble with you. And you really don't need to tell me very much about it because you understand what the trouble is, and you know more about how your wife feels than I do since I haven't met her. And as you start thinking the matter over, and delving into your own mind about it, you can really absorb yourself in that effort to understand what is taking place within you when you are having problems, when you are seeking to understand, and *I would like to have you feel very comfortable as you begin to examine those ideas.* Nothing else is really important except understanding your problem, and understanding

Editors' Note: See *Hypnotherapy* for a more detailed examination of discharging resistance via the negative.

how you want to feel, and understanding why you want to feel in certain ways.

Now your feelings may be positive, they may be negative, but *I would like to have you feel exceedingly comfortable about this matter of a straightforward, careful examination within your own mind* about all of these things that are troubling you emotionally—perhaps troubling you in a great variety of ways—and just give your attention to those particular things. And you can select out of all that I say those words that are meaningful to your problem.

Brain Functioning and Psychopathology: Unlimited Possibilities for Dysfunction

The point I would like to impress upon all of you regarding this matter of psychopathology is this: that there is very, very little you can teach people about psychopathology that they are not capable of understanding far better than you can explain it to them. Now that may sound rather peculiar, but I think this example will illustrate my point.

Several years ago I participated in a research project on schizophrenia at the Worcester State Hospital in Massachusetts. A sixteen-year-old boy from a very isolated, rural community was brought in to see me. His parents were illiterate; they did not believe in education; they had allowed that sixteen-year-old boy only to attend the first few grades of school.

Taking the mental examination on this boy turned out to be a most amazing experience for me because he gave me such a rich array of delusions and hallucinations, some of which I recognized from my readings on folklore. One of his delusions was quite comparable to the rose of Central Africa in Frazier's *The Golden Bow*. I checked to see if he had ever read *The Golden Bow,* but not surprisingly, he had not. He told me all about the _____ [end of sentence lost in the recording]. He had to keep his hand in front of his mouth so that his soul would not escape.

"What would happen if you spit on someone?", I asked him.

"I would lose my soul," he replied, "unless you were a friend

187

of mine. I could spit on the hand of a friend of mine, and I could trust him because the spit would be my soul—it would be my life."

I had him draw pictures of men and of women, and then I got out my copy of Princehorn. It is in German, and it contains artwork of the mentally ill. My sixteen-year-old illiterate patient had drawn pictures of men and women that looked very similar to those Princehorn had recorded from his patients living in Germany around the turn of the century. Now my patient had not been born in, or near, 1900; and he certainly could not read the German language; in fact, he could not read any language. Yet he had the most completely involved and elaborate delusional and hallucinatory system that I had ever encountered. I was amazed—an untutored, unlettered, sixteen-year-old kid with a highly involved, highly complex delusional and hallucinatory system that I could match with readings from Frazier's *Golden Bow* and from Princehorn's book as well! How on earth did that kid manage to develop ideas as complex as he developed, and to do it all from scratch!*

This patient gave me a tremendous respect for what the human mind can do. All of these brain cells that we have can go into action and produce all manner of permutations, so that you can get all possible varieties of psychopathology. Every time you work with a patient hypnotically, you ought to bear in mind that the patient might do things of a rather peculiar sort, and in a most unexpected fashion.

Psychopathology and Aphasia:
The Amazing Case of Interrupted Words

I don't know how much you know about aphasia, but to begin with, there are various types of it. You all studied English

---

*Editors' Note: Erickson seems unaware that this is exactly the sort of phenomenon that the psychiatrist C. G. Jung used to illustrate his theory of archetypes and the collective unconscious: that the human mind is predisposed by its organic structure to organize experience into certain mental-behavioral patterns called archetypes. See C. G. Jung, *The Arche-*

in grade school, in high school, in college. You know what an adjective is, what an adverb is, what a noun is, and what a preposition is. But how on earth do people develop an aphasia for nouns as a result, let us say, of a cerebral accident? They can talk freely and easily, but they cannot utter a single noun because they have a nominal aphasia. They do not know the names of things.

Then you can have patients with an adjectival aphasia: they cannot say, "pretty girl"; they cannot say, "fat girl," but they can look at lard and call it "fat," because there the word *fat* is a noun and not an adjective.

Now how does the brain manage to do that sort of thing? I can think of one man who had a particular type of arterio-sclerosis. I asked him to tell me a story, and so he started, at about the year one, to give me his own history. The man told a coherent and meaningful story, but it was awfully detailed—he was as garrulous as could be. As I listened to him, I noticed there was a certain pattern in his words, a certain length to his phrases, a certain rigidity in his delivery.

Now I had my medical students with me at the time, [and I saw in this situation an opportunity for an unplanned demonstration]. So, as the patient was in the middle of pronouncing a word—let us say the word *remember*—I clapped my hands or slammed a book to interrupt him and started an argument with my medical students: I bawled one of them out and criticized another, in general creating a violent, emotional situation, to their utter bewilderment. I let the skirmish go on for about five minutes, quieted everyone down, and told the patient to continue. And so he did, beginning with "ber"—[the last syllable in the word "re-mem-*ber*"].

I staged another interruption in the middle of another word, and when I told the patient to continue he resumed the word at

---

types and the Collective Unconscious. New York: Pantheon Books, 1959, pp. 50-53. For a theoretical update, see E. L. Rossi, "The Cerebral Hemispheres in Analytical Psychology," *Journal of Analytical Psychology,* 1977, *9,* pp. 32-51.

exactly the point where I had interrupted him. Then the medical students caught on to what I was doing and they began interrupting him. It turned out that you could interrupt this man for one minute, for five minutes, for ten or twenty minutes, but when he started up again his "needle" was still in the same groove, and his "record" started up at the exact point of interruption.

I also discovered that I could ask him to tell me the time, and he would look at my watch, report the time, and resume his story, again, at the exact point of interruption! How does the human mind do that sort of thing? More amazing, how does a brain damaged by arteriosclerosis do that sort of thing? So when you look at psychopathology, you ought to have infinite respect for the human brain that produces it.

Overcoming Brain Damage and Evoking New Learning via Anger, Provocation, and Frustration: Janet's Pease Porridge Hot

I can think of another case I wrote up in *The American Journal of Clinical Hypnosis.**

Janet could not talk as a result of a cerebral accident. She had lost the power of speech, and the loss was organically based. She had tried to talk for two years after the accident, but all she could get out after fifteen minutes of agonized struggling was a very stammered, "I"; another fifteen minutes of struggle and out would come, "can't"; still another fifteen-minute struggle might force out the word, "talk." The whole ordeal was a horribly painful thing to watch. She would struggle, twist, and turn in so much effort and frustration.

Janet had recovered her ability to walk as well as all other major abilities, but she was still plagued by a thalamic syndrome of pain on her right side. Four prestigious neurological clinics had given her a life expectancy of two to three years. During

---

*"Hypnotically Oriented Psychotherapy in Organic Brain Damage." 1963, *6*, 92-112. In *Collected Papers*, Vol. IV, 283-311.

the two years since she had been diagnosed, she had been lying at home on a couch, smoking cigarettes and staring at the ceiling. She would go to bed at 10:30 P.M., get up at 10:30 A.M., eat a combined breakfast and lunch, lay back down on the couch, smoke cigarettes, stare at the ceiling, eat dinner, lay back down on the couch, and smoke. Her husband and her sons all had tried to talk to her; friends had called on her to try to rouse her; but poor Janet just lay there vegetating. It was perfectly obvious that she was going to die sooner or later. She was losing ground visibly. Her husband finally brought her to me because her general practitioner had recommended hypnosis as a last resort.

I saw Janet on July 1st. I took one look at that wretched looking woman and thought, Why did I ever enter the practice of medicine, because there is nothing more hopeless in the world than this patient! Here was an instance where the psychopathology was organically established, and it followed all the neurological laws. What on earth can you do about that? As I thought it over my feelng was: If I can bring about in this patient enough frustration, enough anxiety, enough fear, enough anger, enough disgust, enough bewilderment, enough curiosity—such that her brain cells have to work in a great variety of ways—perhaps I can then teach her how to talk again.

I developed a rather elaborate plan which I then discussed with her husband. [The first part of the plan required a suitable, full-time companion.] I got acquainted with a relative of Janet's, named Edith, who could talk at the rate of approximately 250 words per minute! Edith liked to talk, and it was awfully hard to interrupt her. I brought Edith into my office and explained what I wanted her to do. She readily agreed, and turned out to be a most cooperative companion.

I told her first that I wanted her to play the "Pease Porridge Hot" game: "Pease porridge hot, pease porridge cold, pease porridge in the pot nine days old." I didn't know all the hand movements that went with the rhyme, so I asked my wife to come in and show Edith the correct movements. Edith began remembering the whole game from her childhood and her delivery of it now became quite smooth and lively. All day long, at intervals of five to ten minutes, Edith would play "Pease Porridge Hot" with Janet, and Janet would have to sit there or stand there and go through that game. Can you imagine how disgusting and frustrating and distressing it is to be interrupted and made to play a silly, ridiculous game—no matter what you were in the middle of doing—every five to ten minutes throughout the entire day! And I had made Janet promise me ahead of time that she would do anything and everything I instructed her to do. I made it perfectly clear that my word was absolute law, and that she was to obey every instruction, however unfathomable, that I gave her if she were to learn to talk again.

Edith played "Pease Porridge Hot" with Janet endlessly. Janet would be taking a shower and Edith would step into the shower and play, "Pease porridge hot, pease porridge cold," slapping and patting her hands appropriately; Janet would be taking a bath and Edith would come in, sit on the edge of the tub, and chant, "Pease porridge hot, pease porridge cold . . ."; Janet would be in the middle of eating dinner, and Edith would break in with more "pease porridge hot." Edith found the most outrageous times to interrupt Janet, and poor Janet would have to play that game, all the while resenting it horribly.

Now as soon as Janet got in a sufficiently resentful state, a rather intensely resentful state, I had Edith introduce the next move. Have you ever listened to a stutterer, and felt your tongue tangle up and your lips twist and turn and your whole body stiffen and agitate as you listen to that chap try to get those words out? Edith now began stuttering the "Pease Porridge Hot" rhyme! And poor Janet was so utterly resentful, so completely and thoroughly resentful. Janet knew Edith did not stutter normally, but Edith was marvelous at linguistics. She could stutter in the most agonizing, authentic fashion imaginable, until at last Janet would explode: "HOT!" She just couldn't help herself. She was so resentful and so distressed that all the muscles of her body started responding to that aggravation. Well, it wasn't long before Janet was saying "pease," and she was saying "porridge," and she was saying "hot."

At this point I again had Edith alter the game plan. Edith would awaken Janet in the morning and ask, "Would you like eggs and toast and bacon and coffee for breakfast?" And Janet, who *dis*liked iced coffee and iced tea, would nod her head very happily at the proposed menu. Janet would take her shower and dress and come out to have that nice breakfast, and there on the plate would be, naturally, sliced carrots, the leaves from celery, a raw potato, and iced tea (or perhaps just ice!). And Edith would proceed to chatter blissfully at the rate of 250 words per minute about the delightful breakfast, and Janet would look down at her plate in a most bewildered way, and Edith would throw in: "Remember, Dr. Erickson told you that you would have to clean up your plate at every meal." Janet would struggle and struggle to say, "But—I—don't—eat—raw—potatoes!"

Eventually Janet did succeed in getting out that sentence, but only after she had been strained and forced by countless aggravations. Edith would take Janet out to dinner, hand her the menu, and Janet would point to where it said *potato*. At first, however, Janet had not been able to read. I discovered she had alexia. She would point hesitantly and hopefully, gesturing her hands as if to say, "You order for me." Edith, of course, had previously discovered all the foods Janet did not like to eat; and Edith would cheerfully order all those unwanted foods and Janet would have to clean up her plate because Dr. Erickson had said so. It wasn't long before Janet learned to read, and she could point to the word *potato* and haltingly speak, "po—ta—to." And when Janet pointed to the words *baked potato* [but did not pronounce them,] Edith would cheerfully order *potato salad* instead, which she knew Janet didn't like. In other words, an incomplete effort was not sufficient. Janet could say, "Steak"—you know—very, very, very rare steak—and that is what Janet got, and she had to clean up her plate.

I had Edith defeat Janet in every possible way. When I thought Edith had taught Janet everything imaginable, I had another companion hired. Lois was a sweet, timid, darling eighteen-year-old girl who didn't want to offend anybody; who would have tears spring to her eyes immediately when she thought she had done something wrong. Now I had also hypnotized Lois to reinforce her hypersenstivity and to reinforce her readiness to shed tears. (I had also tried to hypnotize Janet on several occasions, but had succeeded only when I used exceedingly indirect measures.)

I worked out a specific plan with this new, young companion that I thought especially suited her personality in relation to Janet's. Janet hated popular music; she hated loud rock and roll, or really any rock and roll. Have you ever been forced to listen to the same hated music, hour after hour? Janet was forced to listen to very loud and very noisy rock and roll music, hour after hour; and worse, she had to listen to Lois beat time to it—but out of time! There is nothing more aggravating in the world. Janet had to watch Lois beating time, but always out of time, and poor Janet would struggle to tell her to beat in time. So I asked Janet to beat time with her right hand, then with her left hand, and with the right foot, and with the left foot. Then I gave her the involved problem of left foot, right hand—right foot, left hand; and then crisscrossing in that same pattern. Now I did not know exactly what that crisscrossing would achieve; but I did know that she had had a brain hemorrhage, she had had a brain operation, and she now had a badly damaged brain. So I wondered how many neurological pathways had been damaged, [and how many new pathways she could create] : hence, the exercise of crisscrossing, of alternating the right and left feet, alternating the right and left hands, crossing over in one manner and then back, crossing over in another manner and then back. I had her practice that routine endlessly, both in time to music and out of time to music. Oh, the frightful struggle that went on within Janet to do all this!

Next I had Janet dance with Lois. But now Janet could not step backwards. I understood that particular problem myself because it has been very difficult for me to step backwards since I had polio back in 1919. If I am not careful I fall down because something just goes wrong with the management of my legs; I do not know how to balance myself. I checked with Janet as soon as I knew she had brain damage to find out about her walking abilities, and sure enough, Janet could not step backwards either. So I had Lois dance with Janet: I had Lois dance out of step, I had Lois lead, I had Lois follow. In dancing, of course, you do step backwards.

Now I can bawl out anybody thoroughly when I want to, and I'd reduce poor Lois to a puddle of tears by bawling her out in front of Janet for not doing something correctly. Janet was very maternally minded, and she would be utterly furious with me because it hadn't been Lois's fault, and Janet really wanted to tell me off. With that utterly intense anger Janet got to the point where she could burst out with one, two, even three words, now and then. It took me from the beginning of July until the beginning of November to make Janet such an excellent conversationalist!

Janet had learned to read again, but as a result of her alexia she could not spell correctly. After I sent her home I played a dirty trick on her by demanding that she write me weekly letters. I told her that I would read the letter each week, and if there were a single mistake in it I would return it to her for correction and rewriting. Now mind you, I never marked the mistakes for her—I simply returned the letter with the statement, "Write it over," and poor Janet would have to search through the letter to find her own mistakes. That would mean that by the next week, Janet would owe me two letters: the corrected one, and a new one! She worked very hard to read her letters through and correct the spelling errors until finally she had learned to read freely and easily; she could read the newspaper aloud, and read it correctly; and she could write me a letter with not more than one or two mistakes in it.

I used hypnosis on Janet, but only indirectly. After Janet had learned to talk again she would chat with me in my living-room (my office is in my home), and she would chat with my wife and children with whom she was also friendly, and we all would have a most pleasant visit there in the livingroom. But as soon as Janet stepped back into my office her face would freeze, her movements would become stilted, she would sit down in a chair, and she would neither see nor hear anything except me and my voice.

Janet was living in a new home in Tucson which her husband

had built especially for her. They had moved to Arizona from Wisconsin in order to be near me, but Tucson is 125 miles from Phoenix, so Janet could not become too dependent upon me. I went to visit Janet in her new home. She was quite proud of it, and took me on a thorough tour. When I first arrived and throughout the tour, Janet clearly played the role of a hostess with a guest, but when we sat down for the professional interview she promptly went into a trance.

"You know," she said to me, "something happens to me when you start talking like a doctor. Everything changes. Am I in a hypnotic trance?"

"You are in the kind of trance that is going to help you in every way," I answered.

I saw Janet regularly every month for four months until she finally died of renal necrosis caused by taking too much phenacetin for her thalamic pain. She had the thalamic syndrome— right-sided pain. Even a very delicate touch would make Janet wince and tears come to her eyes. This delicate touch did hurt. Janet had a great deal of difficulty. I couldn't reduce that thalamic syndrome too much. I reduced it to the point where her dress, her stocking, her shoe, her clothing would not distress her: so that she could sit down, she could drop her hands in her lap, and so on, and she would not suffer that horrible thalamic pain. She had had the brain surgery in an attempt to reduce that horrible pain, but the surgery had not helped. I had reduced it somewhat, but I could not remove it entirely.

Entering the Patient's Framework to Facilitate a Fractional Approach to Phobia Reduction: The Tall Building Phobia

I have gone to considerable length in discussing this matter of psychopathology. Of course, there are many types of psychopathology that are not organically caused. You ought to bear in mind that the best approach to a patient's psychopathology lies in your own sympathetic attitude.

I can think of one man in particular who came to me for help. He had been in the construction business; he had owned his own firm, and he had built tall buildings, but finally he had been forced to give it up. Why?

"I am afraid to walk down the street because those buildings might fall down and crush me," he told me.

He was reduced to absolute poverty. He simply could not get along in the city because he believed he had to avoid any building over four stories high for fear it might topple over and crush him. So I asked him in the hypnotic trance state to tell me how high a five-storied building, a six-storied, eight-storied, ten-storied building would be, and how far across the street, how far across the block, each building would reach if it tipped over. I explained to him that if a building were, say, 100 feet high, then it would be perfectly safe for him to walk past it from a distance of 130 feet—the extra 30 feet being added to allow for flying debris. Now he could agree to this logic. It made sense to him.

Next I suggested that he map out the various streets and the various buildings in Detroit and calculate what particular distance away from each building he would have to walk in order to feel safe. What he didn't realize was that I was educating him to walk past each of those buildings. He thought I was educating him in the matter of passing them safely, and I was; but in walking past them safely he was first of all *walking past* them. Previously he had not been able to go downtown in Detroit for fear that the buildings would fall on him. But once we had mapped out the city of Detroit so that he could actually walk here and there, he took a great deal of pleasure in walking here and there.

Next we started shading the distances. Instead of requiring 130 to 140 feet of distance for a 100-foot-high building, well, he could walk 139 feet away from it, 138 feet away from it, 137 feet away from it, 136 feet away from it, 130 feet away from it, and so on, until finally he could walk just 100 feet away from it, and do so safely. I also pointed out to him that you can see the building begin to fall, and how long will it take a 100-foot-high building to fall all the way to the ground? Just figure it out, and during that length of time how far away can you get from that dangerous 100-foot distance? So I introduced another element—the time element—and he soon figured out that he could walk 90 feet away from a 100-foot-high building, because that would still give him enough time to get out of harm's way. But what that man was really doing was gradually getting used to the idea of walking past high buildings from increasingly closer distances.

Entering the Patient's Framework to Facilitate a Fractional Approach to Symptom Reduction: 20 Percent Asthma

An example of another type of psychopathology is the asthmatic patient. How accustomed do asthmatic people become to not being able to breathe freely? I can think of a twelve-year-old patient of mine who had asthma and who was very dependent upon his inhaler; he would use that inhaler countless times in order to breathe comfortably while talking to me in my office. I asked him to explain the intensity of his fear. I did not try to convince him that he could breathe just fine; I did not reiterate to him the facts that he was twelve years old; that he had had asthma since he was a small child; and that he had grown up in a constant state of fear about his breathing.

Instead, I asked him to tell me, to help me understand, how important his fears of not being able to breathe were. This was the first time anyone had wanted to listen sympathetically to an account of his fears about dying from arrested breathing. And he got awfully interested in telling me all about the intensity of his fears; about his nightmares of a sudden arrest in breathing; about the horrifying constriction in his chest; about the terrible visions that came to him, and so on. While he was recounting all these fears, he became so fascinated by at last having a good listener that he began breathing more comfortably. When I felt it was safe enough to point that out to him, I said:

"You know, talking about your fear makes it easier for you to breathe, and so I would like to have you understand that some of your asthma is caused by fear, and some of it comes from the pollens, and so on. That is why you take the medication you take.

"Let us begin by assuming that you have 100 percent asthma. Now you wouldn't notice the change if I reduced that asthma by 1 percent, but you nonetheless would have 1 percent less asthma. Suppose I reduced it by 2, by 5, by 10 percent? You might not notice it, but it still would be reduced."

Then I got him interested in this idea that perhaps he could reduce it by 10 percent, by 15 percent, by 20 percent, 25 percent, 30 percent, and so on; and then we started debating what percent of his asthma he was going to keep! Would he keep 5 percent of it, 10 percent, 20 percent, 30 percent, 40 percent, and so on, with the result that this twelve-year-old patient voted to keep just 20 percent of his asthma. He felt that 20 percent was the amount of asthma that was organic in origin. [That meant that he had altered his concept of his asthma almost full circle: from viewing all of it as being caused by pollens to viewing only 20 percent of it as being caused by pollens, and the remainder being caused by his own fear.] He made quite a shift in attitude here that he transferred beneficially into other areas of his life.

You approach the correction of psychopathology by a gradual eradication of it, not by attempting to contest it, dispute it, or annihilate it.

Utilizing the Perversity of Human Nature to Establish or Alter Normal Physiological Functioning

A most important orientation to keep in mind is that you must have adequate motivation in order to discover what a person can do physiologically.

This morning I was reminded of the potential perversity of human nature, and the way in which human perversity affects physiological functioning. I will give you an example. You are at the movies. You feel an urge to go to the bathroom, but you decide you would rather use your own bathroom, and besides, the show will be over shortly. So you sit through the end of that feature, and then another feature comes on the screen and you manage to sit through it, but you still decide to wait until you get home to go to the bathroom. There are a couple of traffic jams on the way home, but then you are used to encountering traffic jams and you get along just fine. You finally drive into your own yard, get up to the front porch—now where is the house key?? That is when the trouble begins, and I think that is the way a lot of dances were invented.

What is the practical application in this example? When I did my medical internship it was with the understanding that I would not, under any circumstances, use hypnosis. I solemnly agreed not to use hypnosis; and was told not even to mention the word.

Many surgical patients will have retention to the point where they simply cannot make themselves function. Well, I have never liked to catheterize patients. I am just naturally lazy, so when one of my post-surgical patients would develop retention I would say, ever so sympathetically, "Well, sooner or later, you will feel an urge to urinate but I do hope you won't get that slowpoke nurse when you push the button." That wasn't hypnosis, but the patient would lie agonizingly in bed, trying to hold back urinating until that slowpoke nurse arrived!

I can think of another example that shows how you can use the perversity of human nature very nicely to alter physiological functioning. One afternoon a patient simply decided that she was going to remain in my office for the rest of the afternoon because, she explained, she found the hypnotic trance so restful and so comfortable. When she announced that to me I told her that I had other patients to see. She told me to cancel them. I told her I would have to charge her for the additional hours. She said that would be fine. Then I expressed my pious wish that she would feel very comfortable, very rested throughout the afternoon, and I really did hope she would not have to disturb herself to go to the bathroom. Five minutes later she was in the bathroom!

People do behave that way. There is the person who tells you how terribly constipated he is; he tells you how much medication he takes, how many enemas he endures, how very difficult the whole situation is. And you get him in a good trance and suggest that he have a breakfast of graveyard stew (toast and hot milk). Then you express the very pious hope that he get to the bathroom on time. Certainly graveyard stew does not promote bowel activity, but the sobriety with which you express the hope that the patient get to the bathroom on time has the effect of instigating proper physiological functioning.

Distraction and Confusion to Alter Physiological Functioning

There are so many different ways that one can suggest proper physiological activity on the part of the patient. A patient tells you that she simply does not have an appetite for food, and you point out that this is Wednesday. Now obviously Wednesday has nothing to do with the problem, and she is going to be rather curious about why you mentioned Wednesday. And after Wednesday comes Thursday. Now that is an impressive, dramatic statement to make, but everybody knows that Thursday comes after Wednesday, so why are you mentioning it? And then the question really becomes, "Will it be on Friday, or will it be early Saturday morning when your appetite returns?" And the patient has to go through all of Thursday wondering, *Will it be late Friday evening or early Saturday morning when my appetite returns?*

What have you done? You have raised a question, and you have set the scene for the patient to reorganize whatever function she has in such a fashion that she does get her appetite back.

Then there is the patient who says, "The sight of certain foods nauseates me, and there is nothing I can do to control that nausea and that vomiting." What can you do? You get a detailed description of what this nausea and vomiting feels like—or of whatever the symptom is—so that you know the full horror of the problem. Having gotten that, you then raise some very interesting questions: "Do you think you can retain that symptom all through the month of February, which is a short month, and all through March? Will it really last until April Fools Day? Will it last past Independence Day?"

You raise any number of irrelevant and nonpertinent questions in a most impressive fashion. What you are actually doing with these nonsensical questions is directing patients' attention away from their fixed and rigid beliefs about *not* being able to resolve certain problems and raising the question of when *will* they be able to resolve the problem they need to resolve. It is a distraction technique; it is a confusion technique; but in that, it is pointing out to patients that they'd better be thinking about the fact that they can do certain things and they can achieve certain things.

You have a patient who tells you, "I have a neurodermatitis and it itches furiously." You want to know whether it itches worse on Friday or on Saturday, and is late Sunday afternoon the worst time of all. The patient knows you are making a searching inquiry, and you really are. It is a meaningless inquiry so far as science is concerned; but so far as body functioning is concerned it is not a meaningless effort.

I recall another patient who had Raynaud's Disease* with whom I used this particular approach about the day of the week and the hour of the day, and so on: "At what hour—would it be at half past two or at a quarter of three—will you get that good, warm feeling in your fingertips?" And we would debate that question extensively; we would go back and forth discussing whether half past two or a quarter of three were a better time to get that nice, warm feeling. Now the patient was in a trance for our discussion, and she knew I was serious about what I said. *Would* she have the warm feeling in her fingertips was not a question in her mind; the only question in her mind was *when* would she have that feeling—at a half past two or at a quarter of three. And it didn't make a bit of difference to me which time she chose. Once I had conveyed that new idea to her it was easy for her to understand that she could get that warm, flushed feeling in her fingertips more and more frequently.

With the neurodermatitis, with the Raynaud's Disease, you wonder about this matter of altering the blood supply: about the cooling of the skin, about the flushing of the skin, about the

---

Editors' Note: Raynaud's Disease is characterized by spasms of the blood vessels in the limbs, especially the legs and the toes. The spasms are initiated by cold and by emotional stress, and result in an aching feeling of cold in the affected area.

202

whereabouts of the symptom—and you really debate all these issues. People have very fixed and rigid ideas about physiological functioning, and if you try to dispute those ideas I think you are going to end up behind the eight ball. You ought to pick an issue that can be safely disputed and that will not interfere with the patient's adequate functioning. That is why I pick such irrelevancies as the month of the year or the day of the week or the time of the day or the color of food to raise as the disputable issue, and *I let the issue of proper physiological functioning be accepted as a matter of fact.* You really ought to observe all of your patients' behaviors and see in what way you can adapt those behaviors to their benefit when they come to you with various complaints.

Shock and Surprise to Depotentiate Rigid Beliefs and Restore Normal Sexual Functioning: The Polysyllabic Couple*

In conducting psychotherapy for functional or psychosomatic difficulties, you ought to observe your patient very, very carefully. You also ought to have an awareness of who you are and of what your own capabilities are; and you really ought to know a good deal about your own personality [in order to utilize it effectively in various therapeutic situations]. I have had lots of people tell me what a nice, soft, gentle person I am. But I can refer you to many medical students who will tell you the exact opposite; I can refer you to many patients who will tell you the exact opposite. I like to change my attitude toward patients in accord with their particular needs.

I am going to cite a case that I have never had the courage to write up and publish. A professor from the nearby university phoned to make an appointment for himself and his wife. I took careful note of that phone call. The man's voice said that because of certain difficulties existing within the total home

Editors' Note: See "Psychological Shocks and Creative Moments in Psychotherapy," *Collected Papers,* Vol. IV, for a discussion of the theory and practice of psychological shock.

situation he would like to have an interview in unison with me. Well, I have had lots of strange requests, and I did a lot of thinking about this particular one.

When this man and his wife arrived for their appointment they entered my office in a most stilted, stiff, and rigid fashion. Even their clothes seemed to be thoroughly starched! Their facial expressions were rigid, they sat down in a very rigid fashion, and I wondered what it all meant.

The man began: "Shall I relate to you as secretly as possible the motivation that led me to seek this interview?"

I did a lot of very rapid thinking, and answered, "As secretly as possible."

The man straightened up in his chair, and his wife straightened up in her chair, their faces froze, and the man narrated. "We have been married for three years. We met at a dance, fell in love at first sight, and within a month's time were engaged. Before we got married we decided to have offspring. For three years now we have engaged in marital union nocturnally and diurnally for procreative purposes with full physiological culmination, [but without success]."

At this point I interrupted to ask the man to repeat that statement. With exactly the same polysyllabic vocabulary he repeated that incredible complaint:

"For three years now we have engaged in marital union nocturnally and diurnally for procreative purposes with full physiological culmination, [but without success]."

I thought that over, all the while observing their extremely stiff and rigid appearance. I asked them a few, simple questions—questions about their dress, where they lived, what their house looked like, what subject the husband taught, and so forth. Every utterance they gave in reply was a polysyllabic definition of what this was, what that was, why this was, why that was—all very stiffly and rigidly uttered. I asked the wife a few questions about recipes, and she talked about her recipes using the longest possible words, and just as rigid and stiff as could be.

Finally I said: "I think that I can remedy your problem. In fact, I think it will be very easy to remedy your problem. There is such a thing as shock therapy. There are several different kinds of shock therapy. You can have electric shock therapy, you can have psychological shock therapy, you can have emotional shock therapy. I am not going to give you electric shock treatment, but if you wish I will give you shock therapy that will correct your problem. I would like to have you think it over quietly, and perhaps you would like to discuss it in my absence from the office. I will return in a half hour's time. That will give you ample opportunity to decide whether or not you want the shock therapy required to correct your problem."

I left the office and returned in half an hour's time. In polysyllabic phraseology the couple explained that they had discussed it at length and finally reached the conclusion that they would accept the shock therapy.

"All right," I began. "With your right and left manual extremities, will you please grasp the sides of your chairs." (Each took hold of the sides of the chair with the right and left hands.)

"Now hold yourselves rigidly, because I am going to give you your shock therapy. Your complaint is this: that for three years you have engaged in the marital union, nocturnally and diurnally, for procreative purposes with full physiological culmination.

"I'll omit just one word in what I have to say to that: Why in hell don't you *fuck* for fun!"

It shocked them. They sat in their chairs, frozen stiff.

"That doesn't quite complete the shock treatment," I continued, addressing the husband. "As you do that *fucking* for fun, pray to the devil that you get her up the creek without a paddle. Now I mean it. Get that straight. I mean it. Go home and do it for fun!"

Three months later the woman was pregnant. When their little girl was born they told me about it, and they also told me the choicest array of dirty stories I've ever heard in my life. Absolutely wonderful. They had had their shock treatment. When you get somebody that utterly rigid, how long would you have to work with them if you used a gentle, understanding, considerate, careful approach? I think I'd still be doing psychotherapy with them if that had been the case. Instead, I shocked them into a state of well-being in just one interview.*

Shock and Surprise to Depotentiate Rigid Beliefs and Restore Normal Sexual Functioning: Eva's Single Treatment

I can think of another example. Eva was engaged to a man in the Army. He was discharged in May, and he wanted to marry her that June before he went back to North Dakota where he lived. But Eva said no, she would marry him in December. He made all of the wedding plans for December, but, come December, Eva explained that she would marry him next June. Come June, Eva explained that she would marry him next December; come December, she promised to marry him in June. She waltzed him around like that for four long years—always promising and then postponing the marriage.

Eva also had developed a terrific phobia for traveling. The only way she could get from her home town up to Phoenix to see me was to have her mother, her aunt, and a cousin bring her in a car—the mother sitting on one side of her, the aunt sitting on the other side of her, and the cousin driving the car. It was a very harrowing experience. I knew I'd better get Eva over her fear of traveling, but I was very sympathetic and gentle with her for the first few visits. Eva developed a liking for me—a good rapport, a good transference—and then I demanded that she come up to see me alone on the bus. I made myself sound so demanding that she complied. Then I demanded that she come up to see me on the train, and she did. Then I told her that this matter of promising to marry her fiancé every six months and then postponing it didn't mean anything to me, but that it would have to be corrected nevertheless. Now she had just gotten a letter from him (this was late June) stating that if they were not married by the coming September he was going to find

---

Editors' Note: Notice the seemingly paradoxical quality of Erickson's technique here: the administration of a psychological *shock* is used to bring about a state of *well-being.*

himself another girl, and that was that. I read the letter, and there was no question that the young man meant what he said. I read the letter aloud to Eva, and then I said:

"This is the first of July, and your fiancé obviously means this, and so I will have to cure you of postponing the marriage. I will do that exactly one week from today, on the 8th of July. Now between today and the 8th of July you'd better think the matter over.

"Do you want to marry this man? Do you want to marry him enough to get over whatever it is that you are afraid of—whatever it is that makes you postpone the marriage?"

She had told me that she had no understanding of why she was afraid to marry her boyfriend. I told her the treatment would not be the least pleasant; that she wouldn't enjoy it—nobody would enjoy the kind of treatment I had in mind; but that she would be cured. I told her not to report at two o'clock on July 8th unless she were willing to be cured; that when she came into the office she was to do whatever I asked her to do; she was to do it silently, keeping her mouth shut; she could regret having come, but nevertheless she had to go ahead and do exactly what I told her to do.

Eva came into the office at two o'clock, hesitant and fearful, and to her surprise there sat Mrs. Erickson. Mrs. Erickson closed the door and pulled the curtain and took her seat. Mrs. Erickson didn't know what was going to happen.

I said to Eva: "Step over there with your back toward the bookcase, but about two feet away from the bookcase, and keep your mouth SHUT. I don't want you to say a thing. I want you to do certain things.

"Take off your shoes." Eva looked startled and took off her shoes.

"Take off your stockings." Eva looked a little bit alarmed, but she took off her stockings.

"Take off your dress." She was actually wearing a blouse and a skirt. She started to correct me, but then she closed her mouth very tightly and took off her blouse.

"Take off your skirt . . . take off your slip . . . take off your bra . . . take off your panties. . . . Now with your right hand touch your left breast . . . touch your right breast . . . touch your genital area . . . turn your back to me and touch your right buttock . . . touch your left buttock. . . . Now put your clothes back on.

"I don't think you will need a second treatment. Your boyfriend lives in North Dakota, and I think you had better buy a ticket and go up and tell him that you will marry him this month. I am quite sure a second treatment will not be necessary."

She bought that ticket. She went up and told him. He came down to Arizona and they were married in her home town that month. Eva has sent me a Christmas card each year with a picture of the latest child. She has four now.

I gave her a rough treatment. It was shocking treatment. It was an unorthodox treatment, but what are you going to do with a nice, pretty girl who keeps postponing marriage in such a hideous way, who obviously is in love, who is too timid and too shy ever really to talk to you, and who has such a phobia for traveling. She had a boyfriend living in North Dakota; she didn't have much money; she couldn't be in therapy for a long time. Therefore, I used the shock treatment on Eva, and very successfully.

Eva eventually brought in her whole family to meet me. She is very proud of her family. She is proud of her husband; she is proud of his work. And she is completely freed of the domination of a widowed mother, who was widowed when Eva was born, and who reared Eva so that she was just as rigid as could be. I knew that Eva had a rigid personality, and I knew it would take a great deal to break through that horrible rigidity, but once you break through that horrible rigidity you can achieve a great deal. Ordinarily, we think that we have to get at the underlying cause of the problem, [but that is not always the case].

Psychological Shock and Surprise to Depotentiate Obsessive-Compulsive Behavior: The Case of "Salaame Annie"

I can think of the story of Anne. Anne was a student at Wayne State University. She never had managed to get to a high school class on time. She never had managed to get to a college class on time. Anne had entered medical school with the highest of grades. But every professor in the medical school had bawled her out, in one fashion or another, for being fifteen to twenty minutes late, repeatedly, for class. Anne was always late. It went around the school: "Wait until she gets Erickson's class—then we will have an explosion that will be heard around the world!" The other professors knew how drastic some of my tactics were for medical students who wanted to "have it out" with me.

The morning that Anne was to attend my eight o'clock lecture every student had arrived by half past seven. Everybody wanted to see what I was going to do. Anne was there, too. All the students except Anne filed in at eight o'clock. I began the lecture, but I knew the medical students were not listening to me because they were too busy waiting for that door to open. Fortunately, I knew from the other professors what to expect in regard to Anne's specific procedure: It was to walk across the front of the room, down a side aisle, across the back of the room, halfway up the other side aisle, then to the middle aisle and in between the rows of seats.

Twenty minutes past eight the door opened and in walked Anne. Everyone turned to see what I would do. This is what I did [Erickson touches his finger to his lips to indicate silence and then gestures a greeting in an exaggerated, Middle Eastern fashion], so all the students rose. They were as bewildered as could be, and so was Anne, but she kept right on walking—with one eye fixed on me. I most graciously salaameed* Anne, and every member of the medical class salaameed Anne as well, and so we salaameed Anne all the way around the room.

At the end of the hour the medical students made a wild run to tell everybody what had happened to Anne. The Dean met her out in the hall: he silently salaameed her; the janitor met her and salaameed her; the secretary met her and salaameed her. Everybody that met Anne that day did a beautiful, elaborate

*Editors' Note: Salaame is the English transliteration of the common Arabic greeting for arriving and departing, "Ma salaame." It means, "Go (come) in peace."

salaame! Anne was the first one in the lecture room the next morning. That was the end of "Salaame Annie's" difficulty! Several years later Anne came out to see me and she reminded me of what I had done to her.

"It was rather effective, wasn't it?" I asked her.

"Yes," she said, "and it gave me a very special insight. It taught me that you do not have to know the underlying cause of an obsessive-compulsive complaint such as I had. All you did was to render my obsessive-compulsive behavior so ridiculous that I didn't dare to show it ever again. I felt so relieved that I didn't have to be late for class."

I asked her how she was getting along in general. She was fine.

"Any aftereffects from that horrible treatment that I gave you?" I asked.

"No," she answered, "but I learned to laugh to myself about it afterwards because, really, you know it was funny. I knew what the others had said about you causing a big explosion, and I knew you couldn't make any bigger explosion than the Dean had made on some occasions, but when you did it that way it left me so helpless that I couldn't keep that obsessive-compulsive behavior going. I didn't really have a need for it. I did have a need to get to the classroom on time, and I learned to enjoy it."

I cite this story as an instance where there was no effort made, as far as the patient knew, to do therapy; no effort to unearth underlying causes. Anne had a long-established negative behavior pattern that had gone on all through high school, all through college, all through medical school. And just that one, appalling incident served to correct her problem.

I have employed that sort of a surprise technique more than once with patients. Once you break through rigid, fixed patterns of behavior patients are forced to reorient; they are forced to pick up the pieces, to put them together; and they are forced to function in a totally different way. It is so awfully important for you to be aware of these dynamics. I cite these particular examples because they are much more dramatic than being soft and gentle and nursing a patient along slowly and patiently.

210

When you nurse a patient along slowly you can only try here and there to insert something that will put a crack in the fixed and rigid behavior, [but when drastic measures are called for you can fracture an entire pattern of negative behavior with one well-timed, well-executed technique].

I confronted poor Eva with a drastic measure. I gave her one week to think it over, to get set; I gave her no specific warning other than to tell her that she would regret showing up for her two o'clock appointment, but that *she would be cured;* she would regret coming, but *she would be cured;* it wouldn't be pleasant, it wouldn't be agreeable; but *she would be cured.* I gave her a whole week to let that ideation ferment in her mind so that she would be in a state of preparation to receive something that she believed would cure her, and it did. She had a week's worth of dread, curiosity, and full expectation that she was going to be cured.

Creating Expectations of Cure: Structuring Psychological Shock: Authoritarian Approaches

I think it is essential to let your patients know that they are going to be cured; that there is no doubt in your mind about it whatsoever. You are so utterly confident, and you let them know that a cure is going to take place within them. And when they have something awfully unpleasant wrong with them, let them have a little emotional agony before they are cured. I thought Eva was entitled to a lot of emotional agony, so I gave her a week's emotional agony, but with the promise of cure.

As to the professor and his wife, I let them sit there rigid and stilted and fearful as could be. What kind of a psychological or emotional shock would I give them? They'd better take a full half hour to think that over, and I would leave them alone to do it. It must have taken a tremendous amount of courage for them to come into my office and disclose their complaint to me. They phrased it in such wonderful language; they phrased everything they said in such wonderfully horrible language. Then I set up a situation of emotional dread for them in which they could expect something utterly devastating to

211

occur. Why not thoroughly fracture their particular problem; why not leave them without any possibility of saying, ever again, "For procreative purposes only . . ."? Why not rob them entirely of that phraseology [by shocking them out of it]?

Sometimes you can set things up in a very gentle, courteous, soft way; other times you can be rather rough. Certainly with Anne I was an absolute gentleman in salaaming her, but with the exact opposite effect: her neurosis was insulted! There was nothing insulting about an entire class of students courteously salaaming Anne as a person, but it *was* insulting to salaame Anne as an obsessive-compulsive neurotic.

Fortunately, she had the name of Anne, so "Salaame Annie" fitted in a very nicely as a beautiful poem. Touching my fingers to my lips indicating that there should be silence when Anne entered the room led everybody to be silent. Then the next day when the students found Anne the first one in her seat there was no opportunity for anybody to salaame her—no occasion. The occasion had been removed by Anne arriving on time, and so the therapeutic measure was destroyed as soon as it became effective.

When you structure a psychological and emotional situation for patients, try to structure it in a way that allows them to respond to the situation, and yet not to look back upon it as something that can happen to them again. I told Eva that I was quite sure she wouldn't need to return for another session. She had better buy that ticket to North Dakota, and she had better get acquainted with her fiancé's family. And, of course, she didn't dare have a phobia for traveling out of state at this point! I set it up in such a fashion that it would not be necessary for her to strip for me again.

Nothing in marriage could be worse than what I had put Eva through in my office. I was dictatorial, matter-of-fact, autocratic, authoritative; but I used the proper terms, and I simply had her do certain things—identify the parts of her body, touch the parts of her body, and dress again.

What had Eva's fears been? Certainly consummating her marriage would be infinitely less painful than the ordeal she had endured in the presence of Mrs. Erickson and myself. (Having Mrs. Erickson present with her face rigidly frozen didn't help much to ease Eva's experience!) And, sure enough, Eva volunteered the information that her wedding night had been most enjoyable.

The Startle Technique to Facilitate Open-Mindedness, Inner Search, and New Understanding: Visual Hallucinations

I try to meet my patients' needs at a gentle level, at a harsh level, at whatever level they want their needs met at. I can think of one woman who demonstrated this idea to me very nicely. Upon entering my office, she remained standing and announced: "I have seen every doctor in town, and every one of them was so nice and sweet and dear to me; they were all so kind, they all tried to be so helpful, and every one of them failed to help me."

"Well," I responded, "the doctors who treated you nicely and gently and kindly failed utterly, and now you are in here to see me, so shut up, sit down in that chair, close your mouth, close your eyes, relax completely, and go deeply asleep!" And she did.

What was I using?—a startle technique, just nothing but a startle technique. There is the startle technique whereby you slap the person's jugular area—a quick blow to the neck—and that will induce hypnosis; but I don't think it is a good approach. Then you also can take a person who is standing stiffly, let him fall backwards rapidly, catch him at the last moment in the fall, tell him to sleep deeply, and he will go into a trance state—but it is a rather frightening trance state.

I prefer a psychological startle technique wherein the patient wonders, *What is he driving at?* Here, the mind is wide open for new understandings. I am thinking of a particular example. I was lecturing and giving a demonstration at the Philadelphia State Hospital. Out of the vast audience there was not a single volunteer, so I asked a student nurse to come forward. She came forward, saying, "But you are not going to hypnotize me. I'll come forward; I will do anything you want; but I am not going to be hypnotized."

"Is that because you want to be contrary?" I asked her. "Or

is it because you don't want to go into a trance in front of an audience? Or is it that you simply do not understand what hypnosis is? Do you think I would be lecturing here if hypnosis were harmful in some way?"

"No," she answered, "I think it is fine for you to lecture here, but I guess I am just contrary and don't want to be a volunteer subject."

"All right," I said. "Tell me, does that picture over there on that wall belong to a friend of yours?"

She looked at the picture—of course, there was no real picture—and said, "Yes." [She was so surprised by my question that she did not have time to resist; instead, she complied with my cue and produced a completely unexpected visual hallucination.]

The startle technique is simply a matter of asking patients to think about something or to do something that leaves their minds wide open. What is the idea? You've got them searching for an understanding, which is precisely what psychotherapy is about—accepting new ideas and new understanding. As I mentioned this morning, "Should that symptom be resolved on Wednesday? No, today is Wednesday, and tomorrow is only Thursday, but will it happen on Friday?"

Psychological Shock and Questions to Open the Mind: Utilizing Religious Beliefs with Angina Symptoms

I can cite another example. A man was having from ten to twenty anginal attacks every day, and his cardiologist told me: "The man has a damaged heart, but there is no excuse for all those anginal attacks. He is just scared to death, and he is going to kill himself worrying."

When the man came to me for psychotherapy, I used a startle technique of a rather gentle variety on him. Instead of undertaking any type of formal psychotherapy, I decided to utilize the man's own background: I knew from his cardiologist that he was an orthodox Jew, and was very devout in the practice of his religion.

214

As he entered my office and took a seat, I began commenting about how the world is going to the dogs these days; about how it isn't as it was in the good old days when I was a youth; about how there are too many youngsters today who neglect the teachings of their forefathers. Then I launched into a long harangue on the subject of living up to one's faith and practicing it diligently; and somehow or other into that harangue I managed to slip in the idea that if one were Jewish, and it were sunset on a Friday evening, one really ought to give one's full attention to one's religious beliefs and not waste one's energies on other matters.

The man had no anginal attacks on Friday evening, or all day Saturday. He did have one on Sunday. He came in to me on Monday and I explained to him that it was possible to skip anginal attacks; that I thought he could skip them again next Friday, *but why wait until next Friday?* He was so startled by that question—But why wait until next Friday?—that his mind was wide open. Yes, why wait! I had opened his mind by demonstrating something that he had not understood previously. Why would I harangue about religion when I am not Jewish, and yet talk about his sabbath on Friday evening after sunset and Saturday up until sunset? I was giving him an idea; I was opening his mind to the possibility of meditating and devoting his energies to his religious beliefs instead of to his anginal attacks. I said nothing about extending that shift in energy to Sunday or Monday until he returned for a second visit, [by which time he had much success already under his belt].

Psychotherapy: Adapting to Patient Needs

This matter of psychotherapy requires your appreciation and appraisal of the workings of the human personality. You really must learn to appraise every little bit of the human personality and to appraise every kind of available behavior. Then you must adapt your own behavior to the patient's needs on the basis of your appraisal. If you can't adapt to a particular patient's needs then send that patient elsewhere with your blessing. It is inevitable that you will meet patients you simply cannot adapt to. I have told a number of patients that although I would like to work with them, that I think another therapist could do a better job, and that I am interested in having them secure the best possible aid. With this kind of approach to referring patients, they can then go to other therapists with the idea that they are going to get the exact help they really need. They also appreciate the fact that I am intelligent enough to recognize my own limitations, intelligent enough to recognize their needs, and intelligent enough to refer them to the right therapist.

PART IV

AN INTRODUCTION TO THE STUDY AND THE APPLICATION OF HYPNOSIS IN PAIN CONTROL*

Utilizing Hypnosis to Evoke Psychological, Physiological, Neurological, and Somatic Learnings

I very seldom give a formal speech. I don't think I have read a speech to an audience for a good many years, but tonight I would like to follow my typewritten copy. Why? Because the topic I want to discuss is exceedingly complex, and it was a painstaking job to organize the material into a coherent and easily comprehensible presentation. I would entitle the topic of tonight's address: "An Introduction to the Study and the Application of Hypnosis to Pain Control."

To begin with, hypnosis is ordinarily the communication of ideas and understandings to a patient in such a fashion as to maximize his receptivity to what is presented and thereby motivate him to explore his own body potentials toward the control of his psychological and physiological responses. The average person is unaware of the extent to which his capacities and his accomplishments have been learned through the experiential conditionings of his body behavior via his life experiences. For most people, pain is an immediate, subjectively negative sensation, all-encompassing of attention, utterly distressing to experience, and, to the best of their beliefs and understandings, completely uncontrollable by the victims, themselves. Yet, as a result of the experiential events of our lives, we all have built up within our own bodies certain psychological,

*Seminar given in Seattle, Washington, May 21-23, 1965, Section 2.

217

physiological, and neurological learnings, associations, and conditionings that make it possible to control and even abolish pain.

One need only reflect on severely crucial situations of tensions and anxieties to realize that the severest of pain vanishes when the focusing of the sufferer's awareness is compelled by other stimuli of a more intense or life-threatening nature. From everyday experience, one can think of the mother suffering extremely severe pain to the point where she is all-absorbed in her pain experience. Yet, she forgets it without effort and without intention when she suddenly sees her infant dangerously threatened or seriously hurt. One can think of men in combat, seriously wounded, but who do not discover their injuries until hours later when the attack has ceased. There are numerable such examples common to medical experience.

The abolition of pain also occurs in daily life situations where pain is taken out of the awareness by compelling stimuli of another character. The most common examples are the toothache forgotten on the way to the dentist's office and the headache lost in the suspenseful drama portrayed in the cinema. By such experiences as these in the course of a lifetime, be they of minor or major significance, the body learns a wealth of unconscious psychological, emotional, neurological, and physiological associations and conditionings. These unconscious learnings, repeatedly reinforced by additional life experiences, constitute the source of the potentials that can be employed through hypnosis to control pain intentionally, and without resorting to drugs.

Pain as a Construct: Temporal Considerations in Immediate Pain: Past, Present, and Future Memories and Expectations

While pain is a subjective experience with certain objective manifestations and accompaniments, it is not necessarily a solely conscious experience. Pain occurs without our conscious awareness in states of sleep, in narcosis, and even under certain types of chemoanesthesia, as evidenced by the objective accom-

218

paniments demonstrated by experimental hypnotic exploration of patients' past experiences.* But because pain is primarily a conscious, subjective experience with all manner of unpleasant, threatening, and even vitally dangerous emotional and psychological significances, it can be approached by the use of hypnosis—sometimes easily, sometimes with great difficulty. And, interestingly enough, the extent of the pain is not necessarily a factor in the ease or difficulty of approach to it.

In order to make use of hypnosis in dealing with pain, one needs to look upon pain in a most analytical fashion. Pain is not a simple, uncomplicated, noxious stimulus. On the contrary, it has many temporal, emotional, psychological, and somatic significances. It is a compelling, motivating force in life experiences. It is the basic reason for seeking medical or dental aid. Who would bother to see a physician or a dentist if he didn't hurt? *Pain is a complex—a construct—composed of past remembered pain, of present pain, and of anticipated pain in the future.* Thus, immediate pain is augmented by past pain and enhanced by the future possibilities of pain. The immediate, painful stimuli are only a central third of the entire experience.

Nothing so much intensifies pain as the fear that it will be present on the morrow; it is likewise intensified by the realization that the same or similar pain was experienced in the past, and this memory, together with the immediate pain, render the future even more threatening. Conversely, the realization that the present pain is a single event which will come definitely to a present ending serves greatly to diminish the pain, again because pain is a complex, a construct. The temporal aspects in pain which make it a multidimensional experience render it more readily vulnerable to hypnosis as a successful treatment modality than if it were an experience confined solely to the present moment.

There is the example of the cancer patient who knows that

*See D. Cheek, "Unconscious Perceptions of Meaningful Sounds during Surgical Anesthesia as Revealed under Hypnosis." *American Journal of Clinical Hypnosis,* 1959, *1,* 103-113.

yesterday, every 20 minutes, he had severe pain; he knows that today, every 20 minutes, he is going to have severe pain; he knows that tomorrow, every 20 minutes, he will have severe pain. So *at the moment he is experiencing the present pain he also is remembering the past pain as well as anticipating tomorrow's pain: The pain of the moment is thus only the central third of the total pain experience.* If you can do something about the patient's past pain, he won't be able to add that negative memory to the present; and if you also can do something about his future pain, he won't be able to add that negative expectation to the present. [You've taken care of two-thirds of the total pain complex.]

Habitual Aspects of the Pain Experience: Neutral Sensations Made Painful by Association

Another consideration to bear in mind in analyzing your patients' experiences of pain is the matter of habit. Long, continued pain in one area of the body may result in a habit of interpreting all sensations in that area as painful. For example, a person who has recovered from *tic douloureux* [a painful twitch] may still continue to feel pain. All sensations in the newly healed area—the slightest touch, a minor change in temperature—formerly had caused the person much pain, and so he developed a habit of interpreting all stimuli in that area as painful. The original pain may be long gone, but the recurring experience of that original pain leads to habit formation that may, in turn, lead to further, painful, somatic disorders.

Pain is a protective somatic mechanism. It motivates the patient to protect his painful area, to avoid noxious stimuli, and to seek aid. Because of the subjective nature of the pain experience, however, a person develops psychological and emotional reactions to it that eventually result in psychosomatic disturbances: the protective mechanism, in short, has been unduly prolonged. A person with a severe backache will put his muscles into a spasm and then continue that spasm long after the original pain has ceased. The spasm itself becomes painful, and so the backache continues. These psychological and emotional reactions that result in further psychosomatic disturbances are amenable to modification and treatment through the use of hypnosis.

Iatrogenic Health: The Converse of Iatrogenic Disease

Of a somewhat similar character are iatrogenic disorders and diseases arising from the physician's poorly concealed distress over his patient's condition. Iatrogenic illness has a most tremendous significance because the very fact that there can be psychosomatic disease of iatrogenic origin means that the converse is also true: iatrogenic health is fully possible, and it is obviously of far greater importance to the patient. I have always wondered why so many people in the medical profession write about iatrogenic disease, and then speak and write so bitterly against the use of suggestion for health and well-being.

Psychological Frameworks of Pain: Varying Attributes Providing Varying Opportunities for Hypnotic Intervention

To understand pain still further you must realize that it is a neuro-, psycho-, physiological complex characterized by various understandings of tremendous significance to the sufferer. It is precisely for this reason that pain as an experience is amenable to hypnotic treatment. Because pain varies in nature and intensity, it acquires many and varying secondary meanings to the individual in the course of a lifetime, and this, in turn, results in widely varying interpretations of it. Thus the patient may regard his pain in temporal terms—experiencing it as transient, recurrent, persistent, acute, chronic; or he may regard it in emotional terms—finding it irritating, troublesome, all-compelling, incapacitating, distressing, depressing, intractable, vitally dangerous; or he may regard it in terms of sensations—experiencing it as dull, heavy, draggy, sharp, cutting, twisting, burning, nagging, stabbing, lancinating, biting, cold, hot, hard, grinding, throbbing, gnawing, and a great wealth of other adjectival terms.

It is awfully important to have your patient describe his pain in his own words, and to have him describe it fully. As the therapist, you should be careful not to overlook any of the adjectives that your patient uses, because you will need every one of those adjectives in order to use hypnosis successfully. *The different interpretations of the pain experience are of marked importance in determining an effective hypnotic approach to the problem of lessening pain in your patient: each interpretation leads to differing psychological frameworks—to varying ideas and associations—and therefore offers special and unique opportunities for hypnotherapeutic intervention.*

A patient who interprets his subjective pain experience in terms of various qualities and sensations is thereby providing a multitude of opportunities to the hypnotherapist to deal with that pain. To consider a total approach to pain is possible; but much more feasible is, first, the utilization of hypnosis in relation to minor aspects of the total pain complex, after which you extend its use in relation to the increasingly distressing qualities. Thus, the minor successes lay the foundation for the major successes. In addition, the understanding and cooperation of the patient is much more easily elicited for further hypnotic work once he has already experienced a minor success in altering his own pain. Bear in mind that any hypnotic alteration of a single interpretive quality of the pain sensation serves to effect an alteration of the total pain complex.

Division and Reinterpretation of the Pain Experience—"Divide and Conquer"

I can think of the 83-year-old physician whom I treated for the pain of his carcinomatosis. He described his pain as sharp, as lancinating, as stabbing, as cutting, as burning. He also described a heavy, dragging pain—a heavy, dragging, throbbing pain. Now which pain would I approach first? I chose the heavy, throbbing, dragging pain, because the first thing I wanted to do was to teach that man what relaxation is in hypnosis. And what is relaxation? Relaxation is a feeling of inertia—an unwillingness to move. Your legs are too heavy to lift, your arms are too heavy to move, you feel too relaxed for movement of any kind; and along with that relaxation you get a feeling of warmth—a feeling of rosy, comfortable warmth that goes right along with that feeling of relaxation.

Consider how you feel after a good night's sleep, lying in your bed fully rested, and yet it is so nice to lie there and really enjoy just being in bed. Your legs are heavy, your arms are heavy, your whole body is heavy; and you certainly don't feel like jumping up and putting your feet on the floor and getting on with the day.

I found out what my patient meant by the word *throbbing,* and that it was a periodic throbbing—in other words, a rhythmic throbbing. So I could say, "Your legs are getting more relaxed . . . relaxed . . . relaxed," and I could use the rhythm of his throbbing pain for the rhythm of my intonations about relaxation. So I conditioned the throbbing of his pain to the rhythm of my voice pronouncing the word *relaxed,* thereby taking that heavy, dragging, throbbing pain and turning it into a heavy, warm, relaxed feeling in his legs. That was a much desired change for my patient, and I no longer had a doubting Thomas on my hands. He knew that I could do something about his pain because he had subjectively experienced the loss of that heavy, dragging pain. (His illness was severe enough to confine him to bed, so he could well afford to have heavy, relaxed, warm, and comfortable legs.)

Next I could address this matter of the lancinating pain, the stabbing pain, the cutting pain, and the burning pain. I asked my patient to tell me whether I should take care of the cutting pain next—or should it be the burning pain, or the hard, cold pain, or the lancinating pain? What does the patient do in response to such a question? He immediately divides his pain experience, psychologically, into a great variety of separate kinds of pain, and then he asks me to take care of the cold pain, the hard pain, the burning pain, the biting pain, the grinding pain; and I can discuss each variety of pain and offer appropriate hypnotherapeutic suggestions for alleviation.

From Kissable to Homely, and Vice Versa: Dissection to Reverse Apparent Realities

It is much easier to communicate ideas and understandings about pain once you have dissected the total subjective experience. Another example of what happens when you dissect an experience is this: A pretty girl is very, very delightful to kiss. Now you can look at that pretty girl and note how you would really like to kiss her—but you also notice upon close inspection that she lacks a widow's peak so that her hair line is really a bit high; you notice her eyebrows are just a little bit too heavy; her ears stick out a bit too much; her nose is slightly too long; her upper lip is a bit too short; the lower lip is clearly too heavy. Who wants to kiss her now! You have dissected away all the "kissableness" of that girl.

One night I had used this exact illustration in a talk before a medical group. Then I went to the airport to catch my plane, and in walked the homeliest girl I think I had ever seen. I looked at her and thought of what I had said to the medical audience about a kissable girl, and of what I had done to that kissable girl. So I looked at the homely girl, and do you know she had the loveliest widow's peak; she had naturally arched eyebrows; she had a starry look of happy expectancy in her eyes; she had a very finely chiseled nose. I sat there looking at her nose, noting that she had an absolutely perfect Cupid's bow—a natural, beautifully shaped, Cupid's bow. Even her mouth was the right size, and my, wasn't she kissable!

It is the same principle. When you ask a child to dissect and locate the pain experience so that the biting part of the pain is here, the hard part of the pain is there, and yet another type of pain is over here—the first thing you know that child is analyzing and locating the pain, in all its various attributes, to the point where he ceases to feel it at all. [Divide and conquer!]

Hypnotic Procedures in Pain Control

There are certain hypnotic procedures you can use in dealing with pain. The common medical approach to pain is to try to abolish it completely—to get rid of it as a total sensation. But when you deal with pain hypnotically your task is not one of total abolition, simply because it is too easy to fail. Too many doctors try to tell patients to lose their pain entirely instead of letting the pain lessen in one attribute or another; letting the pain lessen in one geographical area of the body or another. You dissect the pain to discover its various meanings to the patient, and then you dissect the pain in relationship to its anatomical distribution. And what if a patient locates his pain in the wrong place? What matters is that the patient believes his pain is over here; it doesn't matter that you happen to know that, anatomically, the pain should be over there. You have a displacement that the patient has furnished you, and you can use that displacement.

Occasionally you can bring about a total abolition of the pain by using permissive hypnotic suggestions—permissive direct suggestions. Every time you tell a patient to forget his pain, you have said the word *pain;* you have reminded him that he has pain. When an enuretic patient comes into my office, he need tell me only once that he wets the bed; thereafter, wetting the bed is never, ever said again—because I can remember after being told just once, and the patient knows that I know it. Therefore, there is no reason for the patient to hear the words *wet bed* again; no reason for me to say, "wet bed," again. The patient tells me his name in the beginning, but do I then remind him that his name is Johnny every ten minutes throughout the interview? I certainly do not. Similarly, I am not going to remind the patient of what his problem is. In handling pain you should be very, very careful to avoid harmful words. One mention of it is sufficient to disclose that you really do know that there is pain; you really do know all of the attributes of the pain; and you do know all of the anatomical distributions of that pain. Once the patient realizes that you know all about his pain—that you know it as well as you know his name—then you can drop this matter of naming pain and naming its attributes.

Instead, you can say the following: "There are certain transformations that can be brought about here. You know how that first mouthful of dessert tastes so very good? And even the second mouthful still tastes good; but by the time you reach the sixty-sixth mouthful, it doesn't taste so good. You have lost the liking for it, and the taste of the dessert has changed in some peculiar way. It hasn't become bad; it has just "died out" in flavor.

"Now, as you pay attention to these various sensations in your body that you have described to me, I would like you to name the particular sensation that you want me to work on first."

What have I done? I have transformed pain into a single sensation. I have given the patient this analogy of eating the dessert, and of the changing qualities in the taste of it. The patient can understand such an analogy, and he can translate it immediately into a lessening of the pain sensation.

Amnesia in Pain Control

There are other psychological measures that you can employ in the matter of controlling pain. One is amnesia. You can ask a person to forget a lot of matters using hypnosis, and the person can forget those matters so nicely and so readily and so easily. And you then can start talking to him about other matters so that he also can forget the pain sensations. You can tell him very simply and very easily:

'One of the ways of dealing with unpleasant sensations is to forget them—like when you go to the movies and get all absorbed in the suspenseful drama on screen, and meanwhile you forget about your headache. You may not remember until three days later that you had had a headache when you went into the cinema."

Analgesia and Anesthesia in Pain Control

Analgesia is yet another excellent technique for handling pain: in it, you produce a loss of pain but not a loss of tactile sensation; not a loss of pressure sensation; not a loss of kinesthetic sensation—no other loss than the loss of the pain itself. You can explain that idea to the patient as a didactic problem, and then let him indirectly begin to apply the new understanding to his own situation.

You can also suggest an anesthesia. Anesthesia may be produced very readily and very easily in certain patients, but it is a rather difficult measure to employ, because when you really produce an anesthesia you cut out kinesthetic sensations, you cut out tactile sensations, pressure sensations—a great many sensations. So unless you are sure of your situation you ought to avoid producing a total anesthesia.

Symptom and Sensation Substitution in Pain Control

Another approach to pain is the method of hypnotic replacement by substitution. I previously mentioned the 82-year-old physician whose heavy, dragging, throbbing pain I reduced to a matter of inertia, to a matter of heaviness, warmth, comfort, and relaxation. I substituted pleasant sensations for the unpleasant sensations. This is a very important technique.

Say you have a patient with a very, very cold pain; and he describes it to you in detail as a very cold pain. Then you bring up the matter of varying degrees of coldness. Sometimes it gets very cold in Arizona—it actually gets down to the freezing point; and I can talk to my friends visiting from Calgary, Canada, about how cold it is, about it being down to the freezing point, and they look at me as if I needed a psychiatrist! And you can talk to someone who comes from Alaska, explaining that 35 degrees below zero is indeed cold, and he will tell you it's a heat wave. That matter of relativity.

You ask a patient to consider all of these factors, and what is he going to do about that cold pain? What is he going to do about that hard pain? What is he going to do about that grinding pain? I want to know if that grinding pain is a rapid grinding pain or a slow grinding pain. Or, I can suggest an addition to the grinding: "If you will just pay attention to that grinding pain you will notice that it is a *slow* grinding pain." I have added my own adjective of *slow* to the patient's grinding pain, and if the patient does not accept *slow* I can slip over to *rapid*

227

grinding pain. Why? Because anything that I do to alter the patient's subjective experience of pain is going to lessen that pain, and so I can substitute a feeling of rapidity or a feeling of slowness for that grinding pain.

I mentioned previously the case of Cathy—Cathy, who failed to develop that horrible, abominable itch on the soles of her feet, developing instead a numbness of the back of her foot; and then developing that annoying, mosquito-like itch at the site of the operation. I wanted to introduce into Cathy's life something subjective that could hold her attention. So I substituted the numbness and the mosquito-like itch at the site of the operation for Cathy's total body pain.

The substitution of sensations is a very delightful way of dealing with patients. You can produce it in children very easily; you can produce it in cancer patients very easily (because cancer patients are usually strongly motivated). The child is in a learning situation. Children are always reaching out for new understandings, and when they have a hurt they want to talk about it and they want to know about it; and so you give them an understanding of their hurt that allows them to handle it in a much better fashion.

Amnesia, Time Distortion, and Displacement in Pain Control

Now, what did I do with the 82-year-old physician who had that horrible, shooting, lancinating, cutting, stabbing pain every 20 minutes, like clockwork? I introduced him to the concept of amnesia and taught him that "you really don't need to remember yesterday's attacks of lancinating pain. It is enough to experience the attacks of lancinating pain you are feeling at the present moment. That is enough. Why bother to remember yesterday's pains, and the pains of a week ago, and the pains of two weeks ago! It seems nonsensical to me. Give your attention to the pain you are having right now.

"And do you really need to remember that tomorrow, every 20 minutes, you are going to have those sharp, shooting, lancinating, cutting pains? I think you can keep very, very busy with just the pain you are experiencing today. You don't have to think about tomorrow. You don't even need to remember that tomorrow you will have further attacks. And once you have had an attack of pain, I think it would be awfully nice just to forget about it, to put it in the forgotten past."

Now these suggestions, while good in themselves, still did not do anything about the sudden, sharp, shooting pains that he would experience every 20 minutes in the present. To deal with this aspect of the problem, I asked him to develop time distortion such that he would continue to experience those sharp, shooting pains, but very transiently. I had timed his attacks, and they lasted from 5 to 10 minutes by my stopwatch; but after he learned about time distortion, the attacks dropped to 5 or 10 seconds in duration. And instead of the attacks occurring every 20 minutes, they now occurred somewhere between every 30 to 40 minutes, and sometimes further apart than that. This was a tremendous gain for the patient. The attack would begin, he would utter a loud scream from the pain, go into a hypnotic trance, open his eyes, awaken, look confused for a moment, and then go on with his conversation—completely unaware of the fact that he had just recovered from an attack of pain that had lasted 5 to 10 seconds!

He had still another very severe type of pain—a continuous, deadly, killing pain throughout his entire body. The question was, What could I do about such widespread pain? I began expostulating on a concept that he could understand: the concept of displaced pain. You can have a coronary attack and later feel the pain of it in your left arm instead of in your heart; you can feel it there very, very definitely, and you don't want to move that arm. I got quite didactic and professional with him in my discussion of displaced pain, and then I pointed out to him that the pain that was killing him was that pain in his entire body. (I'd better say, "the pain that is killing you," because patients need to know that you are unafraid to say the truth to them.) I suggested to him that he just wouldn't give a damn if all the killing pain were over in his left hand—if it were all displaced over to that left hand. He was right-handed, and confined to bed as well, so he easily could afford to put all that kill-

229

ing pain into his left hand; he could easily rest it very, very gently on the covers of the far side of the bed, so that nobody could bump against that left hand—it was so tender and so painful.

The doctor's reply to my suggestion was: "I don't mind having pain in that left hand. No, I don't mind having pain there a bit."

Now what on earth does that mean? It means that pain distresses us, but sometimes there is pain we don't mind as much.* I mentioned that two-year-old daughter of mine who wanted to fight it out with me for the rest of her life before allowing the physician to remove her tonsils. But I swindled her into proving that her stuffed rabbit could too go to sleep just as well as she could.

So my daughter underwent an adenoidectomy, and after the surgery the physician unfortunately asked, "Now, that didn't hurt at all, did it?"

And having a mind her own, she answered, "You're tupid! [You're stupid!] It did too hurt, but I didn't mind it."

A two-year-old child: "I didn't mind it." There was no evidence that the pain had distressed her, but "it did too hurt." She knew very well that it had hurt, but she hadn't minded it, and the 82-year-old doctor didn't mind having all of that killing pain way over there in his left hand. And when his colleagues arrived in the evening to drink a can of beer and reminisce about the past, they would crank up his bed, and he would keep his hand very carefully on the far side so that it wouldn't be touched; and he would drink his can of beer with his right hand, and he would converse and visit with his friends, and have a most delightful time. And up to the day of his death, his left hand had a killing pain in it that he just didn't mind.

This matter of building up a transfer or displacement of pain from one part of the body to another is awfully important. Sometimes you can accomplish it piecemeal, especially in chil-

*Editors' Note: Next Erickson refers back to an anecdote he had apparently related during a previous session, but for some reason was not recorded.

dren. You can say: "It hurts right there, but I think it should hurt here, too, and a little bit here, and some right there." And slowly you direct the patient's attention away from the painful site and over to another area of the body that is entirely healthy: "Now the pain there is beginning to feel better. You are getting nice sensations." With children, though, you had better say "hurt" or "pain," because "sensation" is a word they often don't understand.

Indirect Hypnotic Anesthesia via Dissociation for the Control of Pain: Response Attentiveness and Somnambulistic Trance

Psychological dissociation is another important hypnotic measure for dealing with pain. I can think of the woman with carcinomatosis beginning in her uterus, with spinal metastases, with hipbone metastases; she had pain throughout her legs, up her back, and throughout her body.

I visited her at the request of her physician, who had told me: "Morphine and Demoral and all the known narcotics do not touch her. She is probably going to live for some months, and I would like you to see if hypnosis can do something about her pain."

When I arrived for my first visit she was rather unfriendly, explaining: "I have a Master's Degree, and you want to talk to me about that stage hypnosis stuff, as if that could do something for me. I don't think anybody could hypnotize me, in fact, I don't even believe in hypnosis! I read nothing in college that opened my mind to a belief in that sort of entertaining, mystical nonsense."

The patient's 18-year-old daughter was present, and I observed a daughter who was looking concernedly at her mother, listening intently to her mother, and then when I spoke I observed that she also gave me her full attention. In other words, the daughter showed good, responsive behavior—intense, attentive, responsive behavior. And I said to myself, "Even if I can't hypnotize you [the mother], your daughter here will be a good hypnotic subject."

I asked the daughter to sit down in a chair. I started shifting her hands around to get them in a comfortable position, and the mother watched me. I shifted her hands first this way and then that way, and then this way and then that way. Finally I just forgot, and left one hand in mid air. Since she developed that nice catalepsy, I suggested that she might want to close her eyes, go very deeply into a trance, and forget everything about the disorienting situation she was now in. Well, she developed a very beautiful somnambulistic trance. She had the attitude that if the family physician recommended hypnosis, it must be valuable. She was not concerned about her mother's prejudices; she was concerned only about her mother's welfare, and about any measure that could help her mother, and so she was a most responsive subject. As soon as she was in a nice, deep trance, I began.

"Mother," I said, "you may not believe in hypnosis; you may not believe that hypnosis can do anything for you. But listen to what I say to your daughter."

I turned to the girl. "Jane," I said, "I want you to open your eyes, and I want you to feel yourself sitting over there [across the room] looking toward me; and really feel yourself looking right at me from over there."

Now the nonverbal communication is just as important. I had continued talking to her along those lines—"feel yourself over there talking to me"—and so on, but she couldn't feel herself talking to me from over there unless she were looking in this direction because I was over here.

I continued. "Since you feel yourself sitting comfortable over there, and you are watching me so carefully, notice what I am going to do next."

I slowly lifted her dress halfway up her thighs and asked her to close her eyes. Her mother was looking at me with daggers in her eyes. The daughter closed her eyes very nicely, and the mother saw me lift my hand and bring it down as hard as I could on the girl's thigh. But the girl *over there* didn't feel what I did to the girl *sitting here,* because she was over there! In other words, a very nice anesthesia had been indirectly suggested [via dissociation]. The mother really had expected her daughter to leap up from the chair, because that was a hard slap I gave her.

"Mother," I said, "you like to learn things the *hard* way, don't you. I think you noticed that your daughter didn't wince, but I will ask her if I hurt her."

The daughter replied, "What hurt?"

By this time the mother was getting bug-eyed. "I'm going to give you another lesson," I told her. And I slapped her daughter's other thigh very hard.

"You've got me convinced!" the mother replied.

"All right," I said, "you close your eyes, take a deep breath, and go deeply into a trance." And I proceeded to explain to the mother that when she had her attacks of pain (which occurred irregularly throughout the day and night) that it would be an awfully nice thing if she were to get into that bed on the other side of the room and leave her aching, painful body all by its lonesome self in the usual bed. I got her to understand that.

I happened to be out driving in the desert early one Sunday morning, and I dropped in to see my patient. As I entered the bedroom the nurse held up her hand to caution me, but I didn't pay any attention to her.

"What are you doing?" I asked my patient.

"Oh," she said, "I had an attack of pain coming on, so I took my head and my shoulders, got into the wheelchair, and came out here to the livingroom to watch a television program." And there she was watching a TV program, psychologically, while her aching body was back in the bedroom.

Now the nurse could see the woman's body in the bedroom. The nurse knew I was talking to the patient in the bedroom, and yet the patient would hold up her hand and say, "I don't want to miss this sequence in the program." And I would have to wait until the actors ceased speaking before I could continue my conversation.

In other words, you can use hypnotic dissociation to indirectly induce an anesthesia for patients who cannot learn it by direct suggestion. Just have them move to another part of the room, leaving their pain where they were, and you can get an indirect anesthesia. Don Colcum, an obstetrician, likes to send his patients down to the ocean to watch the waves and the sea-gulls while he works on their bodies back in the delivery room in Bangor, Maine. When it is time, the patients come back from the seashore and he shows them their babies! It is a very simple matter.

Indirect Hypnotic Anesthesia via Dissociation: Betty Alice's Vicarious Learning

For some reason purely feminine, my daughter, Betty Alice, flatly refused to let me teach her hypnotic anesthesia. I knew that she was able to learn it, however, so when she volunteered to be a subject at a seminar I was giving I simply dissociated her and had her sit down in the audience and watch me work on another subject on the platform. Of course, I demonstrated anesthesia on that subject's body up on the platform.

After my daughter came out of the trance, she had a flash of memory about what had transpired. "Daddy," she cried, "you sneaked behind my defenses and you taught me anesthesia!"

"Should I let feminine contrariness interfere with your future welfare?" I asked. "A girl that looks like you isn't always going to remain a girl."

Throughout her first delivery—Dr. Jones was her obstetrician—Betty Alice talked to the audience, to the nurses. She was feeling herself down in Australia where she was teaching school.

Finally, Dr. Jones said, "Betty Alice, don't you want to look and see what it is?" And as Betty Alice reports, she came back from Australia and took a look, and it was a boy. That was her knowledge of the delivery. A perfect dissociation.

Disorientation and Confusion: The Subjective Relocation of Pain to Facilitate Anesthesia

There is another way of dealing with pain that involves body disorientation. I hinted at this technique in the example where the pain is here, and you wonder if it isn't here . . . or here . . . or here; and you very nicely disorient the child.

234

"Let us see, is that pain in your right leg, or your left leg? . . . Let us see, which is your left leg and which is your right leg?"

And you can get as confused as you get the child confused on this subject of where the pain is, and which leg is which.

"And now is it on the outside side of your leg, or is it on the inside side of your leg?" Very confusing!

You can disorient the child fairly easily, but you can also disorient the adult. I can think of the 28-year-old woman who could not write with her right hand and flatly refused to write with her left hand. She had a clerical job, and she insisted on learning to write with her right hand. She had developed a paralysis as far as writing was concerned. So I discussed rightness and leftness, and centrality and dextrality, and so on, until the girl was so confused that she thought this hand was her right hand [her left hand], and this hand was her left hand [her right hand]—because [the left hand] was the only hand that was left to write with!

She continued to write with that left hand that was left to write with for over a year before she got her hands untangled, psychologically. Then she came to me to explain that she practically had two right hands, because she had become so skillful with both hands, equally skillful, and so she was writing with this hand [the left hand].

What was my technique? I set up a body disorientation by teaching the patient to get very confused about the site of the pain, about the part of the body involved in the pain, and about the direction of the pain. You disorient the patient to the point where he simply does not know which side is which, and then you provide him with the orientation that you want for him. If you can move the pain to a place in the body where there is no organic cause for it, then you are in a position to produce hypnotic anesthesia for the pain at its actual site. You move the patient's subjective experience of the pain to the wrong area, bodily, because you can correct it more easily there; the patient has little resistance to accepting suggestions in the healthy area.

235

The Fractional Approach to Pain Reduction:
Losing 80 Percent of the Pain

I previously mentioned the matter of time distortion and the importance of reducing the patient's subjective experience of time. There is another important method of reduction you can use in controlling pain hypnotically, and that is through the slow diminution of it.

I can tell a patient: "I can't take away all of your pain. That is asking too much of me; it is asking too much of your body. And if you lose 1 percent of that pain you would still have 99 percent of it left; you wouldn't notice the loss of 1 percent, but it would still be a loss of 1 percent. You could lose 5 percent of that pain. You wouldn't notice the loss of 5 percent, because you would still have 95 percent of the pain; but you would still have a loss of 5 percent. Now you could lose 10 percent of the pain, but that really wouldn't be noticeable because you would still have 90 percent of it; but you nevertheless would have a loss of 10 percent of your pain . . ."

You continue to diminish the pain–down to 85 percent, 80 percent, 75, 70, 65, 60, and so on. Then you say: "You might even lose 80 percent of your pain, but I don't think that is quite reasonable, yet. I would be willing to settle for a loss of 75 percent." And the patient is going to agree with you, regretfully. Then, "What is the difference between 75 and 80 percent, and sooner or later you can lose 80 percent, and maybe 85 percent; but first, let us settle for 80."

I am still removing pain, but gradually, through a slow diminution of it. I start with 1 percent and continue on until the pain has been reduced as much as possible. As I reported earlier in this seminar, I have used this technique on asthmatics, and with great success. I begin by suggesting that they can breathe with at least 1 percent comfort, with 2 percent comfort, with 5 percent comfort. They still have 95 percent difficulty, but sooner or later I get them settling for 50 percent comfort in breathing and 50 percent loss of discomfort. Then they want to go for 40 percent discomfort and 60 percent comfort, and so on.

Now, these are all the various measures available for dealing with pain hypnotically. You approach pain as a subjective experience. You try to dissect it, to analyze it; you try to get the patient to recognize the various attributes of the various psychologically subjective ways he deals with it; and then you use direct hypnotic suggestion, when possible, or permissive, indirect hypnotic suggestion, for its total abolition. You can use any or all of the following: amnesia, hypnotic analgesia, hypnotic anesthesia, hypnotic replacement or substitution, hypnotic dissociation, time distortion, body disorientation, the reinterpretation of pain, the relocation of pain, and the diminution of pain. You never know which measure will be useful, nor do you know to what degree any one of them is going to be helpful. But you ought to have them all on hand, so to speak, so that you can shift from one to another with ease. You might use disorientation to reduce a burning pain, while a cutting pain seems to call for referral or dissociation. You can never know ahead of time how you are going to handle the individual aspects of the pain.

The Therapeutic Utilization of Resistance: Facilitating the Yes Set; Deflecting Misconceptions

Resistance is a very important phenomenon you ought to be able to recognize and utilize when it occurs in your patients. The patient comes into your office, sits down, and starts shifting in the chair. He certainly is not settling down to a comfortable acceptance of what you are going to say to him. How can you deal with that?

First I ask, "Do you mind standing up?" And he doesn't mind standing up. Then I ask, "Will you please place your weight primarily on your right foot?" He does. "And now shift your weight to your left foot." He does that, too. "Now will you please sit down, and put your hand on the arm of the chair there; now put it here; now put it on the other arm; then put it there. Now, I think you will feel very comfortable."

If patients want to shift their position, why shouldn't I have them shift their position? The point is that *I* have them shift their position; I ask them to shift their position, and I have certainly satisfied their need to shift around. Equally important, I have utilized their resistances, because the more times you get patients to say, "Yes, yes, yes, yes, yes," the more adequately you have started them on this matter of hypnosis.

There is the patient who introduces himself by explaining: "I came here because Dr. So-and-so sent me, but he says that hypnosis is dangerous."

Now that patient really expects me to dispute what he has just announced. [He really expects me to defend hypnosis.] Well, I am not going to do what the patient expects me to do. Instead, my statement is, "Yes, you know, it is something like driving an automobile. There are at least 100 ways of driving an automobile dangerously; maybe more than 100. I have never bothered to try to find out all the dangerous ways of driving an automobile because I prefer just to drive it safely. And that is the way I feel about hypnosis. I like to use it safely, carefully, and gently."

Now, that answers a lot of questions about the dangers of hypnosis without my going into a long, detailed argument or discussion about whether or not it is dangerous: I simply want to use it the way I would drive a car—safely. When you discuss the dangers with a patient, you are really emphasizing the fact that there are dangers. If you simply admit it, and then make it rather ridiculous to debate, you have obviated the necessity for further discussion. [The point is that almost anything can be put to negative or dangerous use; you are not denying or diminishing the potential for danger, but simply putting it into proper perspective—and with the help of a rather straightforward example.]

The Utilization Approach: Converting Resistance into Hypnotically Responsive Behavior: The Need for Practice and Review

There is another aspect to this matter of resistance. You can tell the patient who is resisting: "Naturally, you are unfamiliar with hypnosis. When you were first asked to learn a difficult task, such as roller skating or ice skating, you were also hesitant. When you undertook dance lessons you were hesitant. You showed a certain amount of resistance. Why shouldn't you? Your resistance meant that you were not quite certain you were ready to start the dancing, or the roller skating, or whatever. And now the question is, Are you really ready to go into a hypnotic trance, or shall we wait one, two, three, four, or even five seconds longer, until you really get ready?" And the patient immediately starts orienting in a new direction in regard to his own resistances.

Or I can ask the patient: "How would you best like to show your resistance? Would you like to make up your mind right now that nothing, just nothing on earth, can move your right hand off your thigh? Why not do it that way, and you can really resist any effort to move your right hand off your thigh." I am asking the patient to offer resistance to a movement of the hand. I really don't care whether he moves his hand or not, and yet he is dedicating himself to doing the very thing that I am telling him to do; and he is resisting, and the more he resists, the more he responds!

Whenever you have a resistant patient, I think it is very desirable subsequently to review the particular type of resistance you encountered, and to think of all the different ways you could have spoken to the patient about that resistance. What different interpretations could you have placed on it in a very, very simple way so that the resistance would have become part of the hypnotic induction? You might have said:

"Perhaps you would like to keep your eyes open, and I would like to have you do so as long as you can. Naturally, we all blink our eyes sooner or later. We have done that all our lives, and regardless of how hard we try to keep from blinking our eyes we are really going to blink sooner or later. But you can do your level best to hold your eyes wide open, and that may be your desire, but your eyes have a desire, too, and your eyes are going to blink."

And so you have given your patient the opportunity to keep his eyes wide open, staring at you, but you have also mentioned that his eyes—as if they were something apart from him—are going to blink. He does not realize that you have started a process of dissociation.

Another way to address the resistance: "You know, when you sit in a chair, when you listen to somebody talk, when you are just looking at television, when you are listening to the noises in the street, listening to an orchestra, you shift a foot here, you shift a foot there, you alter your position in your chair. And as I am talking to you, you perhaps will feel an urge to move your hand, perhaps to shift your shoulders a little bit, perhaps to alter the exact position in your chair," and so on. What am I doing? I am asking the patient to shift his position according to learned patterns of behavior. And if the patient is the type of patient who wants to squirm around and keep from going into a trance, I have already anticipated his wants and made his movements responsive to my suggestions. [I utilize the patient's natural behavior as a vehicle for therapeutic suggestion.]

Over and over again, after a patient has left your office, you ought to review in detail every item of behavior. You ought to make notations of the types of behavior, and then perhaps even practice aloud to yourself so that you learn how to phrase your remarks. You ought to mention your observations as if the patient were actually there talking with you, and you ought to practice phrasing the comments that you would make to the patient about the particular type of resistance.

Imitation and Nonverbal Cues to Convert Tension into Relaxation and Establish a Yes Set

A patient says, "I am ready to be hypnotized." And I say, "Yes, and so you are ready to be hypnotized, and I don't want you to strain yourself too much. Let us see, how much of a strain is that position putting on your shoulders?" Meanwhile I am imitating the tensed behavior, and I am thinking, How much of a strain is it to hold that position? And I am thinking about myself, and I can feel my back tense, but what is the patient doing? The patient is beginning to do the same sort of thing; the patient is beginning to feel the tension in his back, the tension in his shoulders, the tension in his arms.

240

As soon as I see that dawning awareness in the patient's face, I can state: "And that tends to make one feel rather tired, doesn't it? I notice that it tires me. And as one gets more and more tired there is a tendency, an irresistable tendency when the body gets tired, for one to think about sleep. And you do think about sleep when you get tired; and you do think about relaxation when you get tired; and as you think about it you relax more and more." Now I drop my arm in a relaxed fashion, and what is my patient going to do?—the same, because we are naturally imitative in our behavior, and we naturally follow examples.

I know that people will imitate, so I am very, very willing to utilize that imitative tendency, only I do so indirectly. I am very careful to appear to be simply self-absorbed—as if I were thoughtfully collecting my thoughts, and so patients feel free to look at me. Why shouldn't they look? There might be something of interest to them. Now I shift my gaze to the other side of the room, and again I seem to be gathering my thoughts, and they again are looking over there along with me. I have given nonverbal suggestions: Look here, look there. They have obeyed my nonverbal suggestions, and the more suggestions you get them to obey the more they fall into the habit of accepting your suggestions in general [the yes set].

Discharging Resistance by Suggesting It: Use of Implication and the Negative

I remember asking a well-trained hypnotic subject to take over the induction of a student volunteer subject. I was using hand levitation on that subject, and he was resisting me thoroughly. It became terribly apparent to the group that he was resisting, so I let him build up that resistance very beautifully. Then I turned to the well-trained hypnotic subject and said, "Art, why don't you take over and deal with this student."

Art said, "I have never induced hypnotic trance, and I don't know whether I could or not."

I turned to the student volunteer and said, "Well, it is obvious that you will be in awfully safe hands."

Art began, "Do you mind sitting over here in this chair?" The student got up and sat in that chair.

"Do you mind putting your right hand up here?", and the student complied.

"Will you look at that window first; and second, will you look at that window; and third, will you look at that window . . . And now, will you just glance at the floor."

I started counting. Art had that subject do about thirty different things, one after the other, and then he said, "And now do you mind letting your hand levitate, slowly at first?"

"Do you mind letting your hand levitate" arouses a negative response, but when you add, "slowly at first"—well, we all like to compromise. And so you build up a situation where, yes, the person can resist; and he can resist by the measure of doing it slowly at first. Slowly at first. And what does that imply?— well, rapidly later! A person doesn't try to analyze what you have said.

Voice Inflection and Intonation in Hypnotic Suggestion

Next I want to discuss this matter of offering suggestions in response to resistance. I think you all ought to write out your suggestions and then carefully analyze them to see what they really mean. For example, examine these [introductory clauses] :

"As you sit in that chair, and as you continue to listen to me . . ."

"As you sit in that chair" means you *are* sitting right there in that chair [the ongoing behavior]. And what about, "and as you continue to listen to me"? Forget the *as* and just notice "continue to listen to me" [desired hypnotic response]. All you need to say is, "As you sit in that chair, and as you continue to *listen to me.*

Then you continue: "Your eyelids will begin to get heavy. Just when, you don't know . . . just when, you don't know. And as they begin to get heavy"—notice I said *begin to get heavy*—"And after a while you will note that they *are getting heavier;* yes, they *are* getting heavier. They are going to begin to get heavy ... they are getting heavy ... they *are* getting heavier."

And so you break your sentence into phrases and you use appropriate voice inflections. Now whenever resistance develops in your patient you ought to recognize it immediately and be able to give a suggestion that is applicable to the particular type of resistance:

"And your foot was comfortable, and then you shifted it so that it would be more comfortable."

What have you done? You have changed the resistance in the shifting into a desire for more comfort, and in so doing, you have given a suggestion for greater comfort. Your awareness of every little thing your patient does in showing resistance or in showing responses ought to be emphasized by the phrasing of your comments: break up your comments and give them different emphases in accord with the type of resistance they are intended to handle.

In the movie last night I hope you noticed that when I talked to the subject in the awake state I used a different sort of voice—a different intonation entirely—that when I wanted her to go deeper and deeper asleep. I altered my intonation very, very carefully:

"And now you will awaken wider awake ... And how do you feel? ... And what is your name?"

Did you hear the shift in the inflection of my voice? You ought to learn to *tie your intonation and inflection to the desired hypnotic responses, and use a casual tone of voice when speaking about those behaviors you don't want included in the trance behavior.* So you speak about resistances in the ordinary tone of voice, and then you can speak in a fashion which evokes the hypnotic response. And you provide a distinguishable tone of voice which the person unconsciously links to the responsive behavior.

Learning to do this takes a great deal of practice, but you really ought to practice just for pleasure and satisfaction. Many years ago I practiced just by analyzing a typewritten account of what I thought I should say. You have the advantage today of using a tape recorder; you can listen to what you said, to the way you said it, and to when you paused.

For example, take the statement, "Now you feel very resistant about going into a trance." And you have paused. What did you actually say?: *". . . feel very resistant about going into a trance."* Patients don't notice it, but what do they do? They begin analyzing their feelings about resistance to going into a trance. They don't consciously hear me say that, but unconsciously they tend to carry out the suggestions. That is why you ought to be exceedingly careful in the operating room or at the bedside to guard your choice of words so that you know exactly what you are saying in the presence of your patients; so that you say only those things that you want your patients to act upon.

Small children are excellent subjects to learn from. They are so literal in their responses and in their behavior. As you speak to them, just pause and hesitate and alter your inflections, and watch them respond so beautifully to the phrases that you are employing. Watch them respond to the hesitations, to the different inflections; and then you will learn the importance of those hesitations and inflections. You gradually will learn to analyze your comments so that you are not going to say anything that you shouldn't say at the bedside or in the operating room.

Discharging Resistance: Shifting the Focus from Contesting to Understanding

There is yet another angle to this matter of fighting resistance. Certainly you ought not to contend with your patient; you ought not to enter into a contest with your patient. So you can say: "Well, I suppose we could really fight it out all day on this matter of whether or not I can put you in a trance, but I really don't believe you came here for that purpose. I think you came here to be helped in some way, and *I would like to understand your problem.* Notice where I am exaggerating my emphasis. I said, *"I would like to understand your problem."* I am saying, "I don't want to fight it out with you for the rest of the day; instead, *I would like to understand your problem,"* and so

244

I have shifted the battleground from one of resistance to one of understanding. The patient suddenly finds himself transported to another level of dealing with me. But I did have the honesty first to concede that "we could fight it out all day so far as resistances are concerned, but really, *I would prefer to understand your problem."* I have cut the ground out from underneath my patient's feet comfortably, easily, and without antagonizing him. At the same time, I have not rejected his request for a duel; and it is a privilege to go along with me and tell me what his problem really is. And so the question of resistance is dropped right then and there.

I could discuss this subject of resistance endlessly. I have found that I often spend more time analyzing a patient's resistance—going over and over it, phrasing and rephrasing what I could say in response—than I spend with the patient during the actual interview. You can vary your remarks so endlessly, and the more you vary those remarks, the better is your understanding of the multitudinous meanings and implications in them.

Learning Psychiatry via Observation and Practical Experimentation

Q: There are many of us who regard you as the prime psychiatrist of our time. Would you comment on where you learned your psychiatry?

A: I learned most of my psychiatry—not in the lecture room, not by listening to some professor—but by listening to my patients, by observing my patients.

In my premed college days, I used to enjoy observing my classmates. While sitting in the classroom I liked to see what I could do to get somebody to do something quite unexpectedly. For example, while my Latin teacher was discussing a Latin lesson my question was: How easily could I look at her attentively and yet get her to start looking over in that direction, because she did see that rapt look of attention on my part, and then . . . [material lost in the recording]. So I experimented in every possible way.

Indirect Ideodynamic Focusing:
Burt and the Car Keys

Let's discuss this matter of directing people's thinking. Several years ago I was sick, and my son, Burt, was home on leave from the Marines. The rest of the family had gone out for the evening, but Burt had stayed to keep me company. And to keep me company he began reminiscing about the time we had vacationed in Northern Michigan. And he talked about Northern Michigan and the quarry, and about the albino frog we had seen there, and so on. All of a sudden I had an urge to ask him, "Would you like the car keys to go for a drive?" For some reason, however, I repressed the question.

The next thing I knew Burt was talking about the trip to Wisconsin from Michigan; about how delightful grandma Erickson's cooking was; about how his brother, Lance, always ate too much chicken and how Lance, in fact, did get sick on the way back to Michigan. And again I got an urge to offer him the car keys, but again I repressed it.

Then Burt mentioned the trip to my brother's farm, and how Allan had gotten so worried: How does the mother hen nurse her baby chickens? And Alice, in the wisdom of her very tender years, had said, "Only mammals nurse their young." She had proceeded to explain very carefully that mammals give milk, and she was very learned. Allan listened to her. Burt and I both laughed about that incident, and again I got an urge to offer him the car keys. I repressed it, and then thought, *Now wait just a minute! . . . Three times I have had an urge to offer him the car keys . . . What has been going on here?*

I slowly put it all together. Northern Michigan—we got there by driving in a car; he mentioned packing up and locking up the cabin when we left—locking up the cabin involved keys; he mentioned going to the quarry, and that involved the car. I repressed it. Then he mentioned going to Wisconsin. That was a long drive, too, in a car. And on the way back Lance got sick, and we had to stop the car—and again I had thought about offering him the keys. And then there was the trip to my brother's farm—another car trip. My conclusion: *Burt has been talking about an automobile all this time. No wonder I have been thinking of offering him the car keys!*

Having completed that train of thought, I said, "The answer, Burt, is NO!"

"Well, Dad," Burt laughed, "you have to admit it was a good try."

"It wasn't quite good enough," I retorted, "because I caught on too fast. You should have been slower and gentler. You stuck entirely to tricks. Why didn't you mention the buying of the bicycle at Ned's where we got the car gassed and oiled? You could have mentioned the bicycle; that would have brought in Ned's garage and gas station. You could have recalled our eating the rabbits that we had bought from Ed Carpenter—I bought the car from Ed. That would have covered up your intent, but you stuck just to the trips. You should have brought in other, less obvious associations to automobiles that would have concealed the meaningfulness of what you were saying, but would still have led me to offer you the car keys."

Burt's response: "I will keep that in mind!"

Sufficiency of Single Hypnotic Response; Subtle Voice Inflections

A point was mentioned to me during the intermission that I want to discuss. In the film you watched last night, one of the subjects said that she didn't know she was in a trance. I asked her why her hand was up. She noticed that her hand was cataleptic and she was aware of the fact that there were other people around. The point made to me by the viewer was that he said he wouldn't have known that the subject was in a trance at all if she had not shown the catalepsy.

What you have to realize is that it is not necessary for a patient or a subject to manifest all of the phenomena of hypnosis to be considered in a deep trance, in a medium trance, even in a light trance. If you can elicit just one phenomenon characteristic of the trance state, you have set the situation up so that the patient can respond to more and more of the phenomena, to more and more hypnotic suggestions.

Another point mentioned to me was the fact that I had instructed the patient to wake up "all over," but the patient did not wake up all over—her hand remained in the cataleptic position. The audience member wanted to know why that was so. I pointed out to him that what I had actually said to the patient was not what he thought he had heard. What she heard me say was: "Wake up, all over." I did not emphasize the last half. I did not say, "Wake up *all over*"; I said, "Wake up, all over." Just that tiny, little change in my voice inflection—a change not noticed by the ordinary person in the waking state—was sufficient for the hypnotic subject. So she didn't wake up all over until later, when I said: "AND NOW WAKE UP ALL OVER." Then she did wake up all over. You need to practice that difference in voice inflection; you need to learn how to break your sentences into phrases.

Trance Deepening as a Function of Patient Needs; Indirect Deepening Versus "Go Deeper," "Go Under"

Regarding this matter of deepening hypnosis, I have found that often too much effort is put into deepening a hypnotic trance. My feeling is that patients should go no deeper into a trance than they need to go. Therefore, I tell my patients the following:

"Now, some patients need to go very deeply into hypnosis, and some patients can accomplish everything they need to accomplish while they are in a very light stage of hypnosis. Neither you nor I know what degree of hypnosis is requisite for you, but I think you are willing to develop that degree of hypnosis that is requisite for you to give your full attention to the therapeutic accomplishments that you need. I think that you are willing to develop that degree of hypnosis that is requisite for you to accomplish the therapeutic achievements that you desire."

I state it in such a way that patients are free to be in a light trance, a medium trance, or a deep trance. I have not made an issue out of going deeper; I have not made an issue out of staying in a light trance; I have not made an issue out of staying in a medium trance. I have simply made an issue out of going as deeply as they need to go. Why should patients go any deeper than they need to go? If you are afraid of deep water, why not swim in water that is shallow?; after all, you can swim in water that comes up to your chin as easily as you can swim in water that is thirty feet deep! Why not let your patients have that same freedom.

Next I say: "You know, in addition to catalepsy, you might, incidentally—and it is not really important—enjoy other phenomena of hypnosis. You can enjoy the catalepsy, but you can also enjoy a feeling of physical comfort, a feeling of relaxation, a feeling of numbness. You can enjoy forgetting that you have feet while you are enjoying being aware of the catalepsy, while you are viewing and reviewing and thinking and analyzing your various thoughts and feelings."

What have I suggested?: a dissociation of the feet. Patients know that I have suggested a dissociation, but I haven't made it an issue. If they do incidentally produce a dissociation they are going to deepen their trance at the same time. But I haven't told them to "go deeper." I really don't like to say, "Go deeper"; I like to say, "Sleep more profoundly and comfortably." I don't like to say, "Go more comfortably into a profound trance," because *to go under* may have bad connotations. *To go* has certain connotations. I don't like that word *go*. How many of us were asked as children, "Do you have to go?"

You try to avoid words that have special connotations of an undesirable nature. Really consider the phrase *go under:* I don't like to have patients *go under* anesthesia; I don't like to have them *go under* an operation; I don't like to have them *go under* hypnosis. You never really know what *go under* means to each particular patient. Why not state it in a way that makes patients feel very, very comfortable: "I would like to have you enjoy a deeper and deeper feeling of comfort as you go into hypnosis."

Your choice of phrases, the emphasis that you give, your use of words—all tend to deepen the trance indirectly.

Hypnosis as a Learning Process; Indirect Trance Deepening via "Extraneous" Trance Learnings

I further explain: "Now really, do you expect to accomplish what somebody else accomplishes who has worked with hypnosis 100 times the very first time I work with you? Maybe you, can accomplish in 50 times what somebody else can accomplish in 100 times; maybe you can accomplish in 20 times what somebody else would require 100 efforts at; maybe you can accomplish in 5 attempts what somebody else would require 100 attempts at. In fact, I really don't know how fast you can learn. I am perfectly willing to have you learn as rapidly as you wish, as rapidly as you can; and I am also perfectly willing to have you learn a lot of things that aren't really important in this situation but which you might like to learn just because of your own curiosity. I am very certain that learning extra things won't interfere with what we are doing.

"Actually, you know, you can eat and watch a television program simultaneously, and your awareness of the television program won't be diminished by your eating. You can smoke without it being a disturbance to your viewing of the program. There are a great variety of things you can do. Your wife may knit while watching a television program; she can knit one, drop one, purl two and not miss a line of the program. Yet, she is executing a most complicated movement that would take every bit of your attention. But she does it so automatically and so effortlessly. And so, while we are working on this particular goal, you can achieve other hypnotic phenomena, incidentally and automatically." What am I asking the patient to do?: to deepen the trance, and to deepen it more and more thoroughly.

The Role of the Conscious and the Unconscious in Autohypnosis: Mrs. Erickson's Discoveries

When it comes to autohypnosis you must make your patients aware of the fact that they cannot do something consciously that should be done unconsciously. Remember Mrs. Erickson in the film last night? I used Mrs. Erickson frequently in demonstrations before psychology classes, before medical groups, before dental groups. I used her so frequently that she became utterly familiar with my lectures; or, to put it another way, she got awfully bored because she knew what phenomenon I was going to call upon her to illustrate next. She would get so impatient that she would save time by developing the particular phenomenon before I asked it of her.

Soon she became aware of the fact that she could hallucinate visually; she could hallucinate auditorily; she could develop anesthesias anywhere in her body—and all with the awareness that I was going to ask her to do it in a few minutes and that she had already done it to save time. Besides, being so bored having listened to me so many times, she became interested in exploring her own feelings. She is a psychologist, so naturally she wondered what the visual hallucinations really were: What were the changes in her vision that allowed her to hallucinate objects that were alien to the particular situation?; what did she do with her ordinary visual reception while she was hallucinating?

As she began studying these matters, she became more and more introspective until she finally realized that she didn't have to wait for me to ask her to develop this or that; she could go ahead on her own and develop whatever hypnotic phenomenon she felt like developing. Then she realized that yes, she could talk in the trance state and, yes, she could think in the trance state: hadn't she just puzzled most thoroughly about the visual hallucinations and about what had happened to her visual receptors? And if she could think, why couldn't she think aloud? So she began to phrase things aloud. She realized that she could actually give a running account to herself, verbally, of what she was doing as she developed a trance state. Next she realized that if she could talk to herself than she could talk to others—she could include others in the hypnotic situation. In this way she learned to go into an autohypnotic trance and simultaneously discuss the change in her feelings, the change in her vision, in her hearing, in her body sensations, in her body orientation; and then she could just simply lose herself in the

251

comfort of the state, or she could work on any problem at hand.

For example, Mrs. Erickson could work on a memory problem. She might ask herself, "Let me see now, what is the verse number of '. . . the moving finger writes, and having written moves on, for all thy tears can't wash out a single word of it'?". Just what is the verse number in that poem by Omar Khayyam? And she could work on that problem by visualizing a copy of the poem and reading it mentally until she came to that particular stanza and its number. She might know ahead of time that when she went into the autohypnotic trance she was going to answer a question concerning a stanza in the poem by Omar Khayyam, and having acknowledged that to herself she could then go into the trance state. But the point is that she would wait until she was in the trance before attempting to answer the question.

The Development and Utilization Stages of Autohypnosis

So many people who attempt to go into an autohypnotic trance say to themselves: "Now I am going to go into an autohypnotic trance, and I am going to produce an anesthesia of my leg because I've got pain there. And I am going into the autohypnotic trance, and I am developing anesthesia." No, that is completely wrong. First you develop the autohypnotic trance, and having developed it, then take over the proper utilization of it. Do not attempt to do both things at once. It is sufficient for you to be aware consciously that you are going to go into an autohypnotic trance, and once you know that you can just wait passively and let things happen.

The insomniac lies in bed and says: "Now I've got to go to sleep—I've got to go to sleep—I've got to get some rest—I've got to go to sleep—I've got to go to sleep—I'VE GOT TO GET SOME REST—I NEED SOME REST!" And what happens? He stays wide awake. He stays wide awake because he is constantly telling himself what he's *got* to do. But the smart person who wants a good night's sleep says: "Well, here I am in bed, and I will wake up tomorrow morning." He just lets sleep happen to him. And surely enough, sleep does come.

If you want to learn autohypnosis you sit down quietly in the chair, you arrange yourself comfortably, and then you say to yourself: "Well, here I am. I have at least two hours, and I wonder how long it will be before I drop into an autohypnotic trance. It ought to be interesting." And then you wait passively, quietly, and comfortably, because you know you will awaken from the autohypnotic trance when the proper time comes. And so you are very comfortable about it. You do not do what the insomniac does. You do not attempt to compel yourself into a state of unconscious behavior from the conscious level.

The Conscious-Unconscious Double Bind to Discharge Doubt and Ratify Trance

I usually assume that patients are going to develop the degree of hypnosis that is requisite. Patients usually sense this trust and respond accordingly, but when they do not, I recognize that they may need a bit more practice because we all have different speeds of learning. And I can point that out to a patient who is a bit disappointed, or who is very greatly disappointed, and who bemoans to me: "I didn't really accomplish very much. In fact, I don't think I accomplished anything." And my statement is: "Well, you know, hypnosis is one phenomenon of unconscious behavior. I wouldn't really expect you to have a full conscious awareness of what you did accomplish, because a good deal of it ought to remain entirely in your unconscious mind."

What have I done? I have placed the patient in a double bind: He's got to recognize that hypnosis is an unconscious phenomenon, and he certainly can't dispute the logic that we can't be consciously aware of what we do unconsciously. And so I let him develop a very large doubt about the accuracy of his conscious evaluation that "I didn't accomplish very much." Instead, he begins to wonder, *How much did I accomplish at the unconscious level?* He begins to question his own evaluation, but he questions it as a matter of deduction from what I said, not because I told him directly to think that way.

Age Regression: The Confusion Technique

Next I want to discuss the matter of age regression. Originally I used the Confusion Technique to elicit age regression. I will give you a rough example.

You all, I believe, had breakfast this morning; or at least it is customary for you to have breakfast in the morning. You had breakfast yesterday morning, and you expect to have breakfast tomorrow morning. In fact, you expect to have breakfast next week. But last week you had breakfast in the morning, and before you had breakfast last week in the morning you had dinner on the evening before that, but before that dinner you had a lunch, and, let us see—last week . . . let us see, last week was May 6th . . . but before May 6th came May 5th, and of course, May 1st always preceeds May 5th, but, of course, April comes before May and you know that April also follows March just as March follows February, and February comes after January, and New Year's Day was such a delightful day, but of course it was only seven days after Christmas. And you are following along, and this happens to be May and we are back to Christmas of 1964 already, but then, you know, Labor Day preceeded Christmas, and before that was July 4th, and we are way back again.

In this manner you keep going backward in your suggestions, shifting this direction and that direction a little bit at a time, until your patients (or your subjects) get awfully confused. They do wait for you to make a sensible, intelligent remark to which they can attach a meaningful significance. And so you say, "You know, this is really a nice day in June, 1940, and it really is."

Q: In the course of regressing patients by the Confusion Technique, aren't you also helping them to organize a good many of the subconscious [memories] that they have at those intervals?

A: At each level, at each date, I'm letting them recall certain learnings, certain memories; I am getting them to think more

254

and more about the past events and the past learnings in their lives. And they are organizing them, and they are paying less and less attention to the events of today.

Age Regression: The Visual Hallucination (Movie Screen) Technique

I later discovered that it is much easier to elicit regression with the following technique: You have the person hallucinate a movie screen, and on that movie screen is a living, moving picture. What am I demonstrating to you now? [Apparently Erickson now demonstrates subtle body cues for reinforcing the reality of the hallucinated movie screen.] My behavior suggests that I am actually looking at a movie screen. It is a nonverbal communication, a nonverbal suggestion; but my behavior—my eye behavior, my head behavior, the position of my upper torso—suggests that I am really looking right at that movie screen and that I am indeed viewing something on it.

"And now a little girl appears from that direction over there, and she is walking happily along. Now she is standing still, but what is she going to do next?" And my subject is aware of my behavior; the subject looks in the direction I am looking and also begins to see the little girl. Of course, my subject is a woman, and who is the little girl she is likely to see? It is the little girl that is herself. Once in a while a subject (or patient) will see another little girl, so then I ask:

"Tell me about that little girl. What is she doing now? I don't see her clearly. I couldn't see that movement she just made . . . What was it? . . . What is she picking up now?" And my subject tells me.

Next I want to know: "You know, I think the little girl is talking to somebody, but I can't hear. Will you listen carefully and tell me what she is saying? Now tell me, what is she saying?" So my subject tells me. I may then add: "No! She said that! And now she is going to do some thinking, and will you tell me what she is thinking?" And so my subject begins to tell me what that little girl is thinking.

Now I ask: "And how do you suppose she feels? Can you

notice how she is feeling? Does she feel the way her feet are placed on the ground? Does she feel the swing moving?" And my subject begins to feel the sensation of her feet on the ground, the sensation of the moving swing.

Where, really, is my subject? My subject is up there in the person of that little girl who is thinking and feeling and sensing and doing.

Next I say: "You know, as you swing up there a voice here beside me can talk to me. And a voice beside me can talk to me." And so she keeps on swinging, and playing with the doll, and making mud pies, and what not; and a voice down here talks to me and tells me what the little girl up there is thinking and doing, because I really can't know those particulars. I can't know what her speech is, what the motion of the swing feels like, what the ground feels like—so the voice tells me. It is a two-stage regression.*

Sometimes I let the subject keep her identity as an adult who is watching the little girl—a very alive little girl doing this and doing that; and then I ask the adult sitting beside me to identify the little girl. And the subject will say: "I don't know who she is. I've got a feeling her name is Elizabeth. Yes, her name is Elizabeth. Oh, yes, her last name is Moore. She lives in Detroit on Martindale Street. Yes, that is right."

Mrs. Erickson's Regression: The Barricaded Street

My wife is Elizabeth Moore, and she used to live on Martindale Street in Detroit. She is telling me about that little girl, and she has dissociated herself from herself as a little girl, but she can tell me exactly what that little girl is doing, feeling, thinking.

Mr. McTear, a professor of psychology at Wayne State University, had said: "There is no such thing as hypnosis; there is

---

*An extensive discussion and demonstration of two-stage regression is presented in "A Special Inquiry with Aldous Huxley into the Nature and Character of Various States of Consciousness," Collected Papers, Vol. I, pp. 83–107.

no such thing as regression." Mrs. Erickson had been one of his students, so I arranged to test his assertion on one occasion.

I had McTear set up the circumstances himself: "All right, make it the year 1934, and have her walk down such-and-such a street; then have her turn and walk down another street, and then have her turn and walk down another street." (I can't remember the actual street names, but he was quite specific.) He wrote all this out on paper for me, and I carefully noted the directions in which he had stipulated that she should walk.

I put Mrs. Erickson in a trance and started her walking down, let us say, Martindale Street. Then I told her, "Now you are coming to the intersection of such and such, so please turn right." Then I had her turn left, then right again—[all in accordance with McTear's directions]. Now McTear practically jumped out of his shoes at Mrs. Erickson's response to the final turn. It seemed he had deliberately chosen a particular day in June, 1934, to have her walk down that last street. (I wasn't living in Detroit at that time, so I had no clue.) What did Mrs. Erickson say as I asked her to turn right on that last street? She said, "I can't—it is barricaded because they are tearing up the street."

McTear had carefully researched his test. He knew that the street had been barricaded during that time period; he had very carefully looked it up in the newspapers. He had made me his innocent victim by having me regress Mrs. Erickson to that previous date and having her walk down that particular street. That is why he drew such a careful map for me to follow—he trapped me into innocently giving suggestions that led her straight to that barricaded street.

McTear did not stop there, though. Next he suggested that I have her walk down the same street so many days later and reread the street signs. And she did. There had been some changes made, and she said, "There is a new sign in place of the old sign." She named the old sign and she named the new sign, which McTear knew had been put up after the street had been re-opened. And Mrs. Erickson was just walking along those streets in her mind, telling us these various things.

I also could have had her watch herself go through all this on the movie screen without any recognition that it was she. I could have had her go through two stages of watching herself, or the single stage of actually being there. Both ways can give you very reliable information.

Two-Stage Dissociative Regression to Facilitate Objective Understanding

Q: In the old days it was the custom in hypnosis demonstrations to have people really relive their age regressions—to be really back there. As a psychiatrist do you feel that there is any great value in doing this?

A: Only in some very special instances.

Q: It's better, then, to have patients look at themselves with the benefit of all their later learnings and perspectives—to help them understand their previous behavior?

A: Yes. I'll give an example. I have asked the patient who vomited at the sight of an advertisement in a magazine to see himself at a previous age level when he could read that kind of an advertisement without vomiting. Then I'd have him see himself with that particular pathological reaction, after which I could ask him to develop an amnesia for it:

"You know, if you look at that person standing there, you can speculate about what the future will be. And what do you think that person really ought to do? If sometime—a year later, two years later, three years later—that person develops a vomiting reaction, what ought he really to do about it? How ought he handle it?"

And I have the patient outline to me the psychotherapeutic measures that should be employed so that he actually conducts his own psychotherapy in advance of the traumatic experience he is going to relive. Then when he does relive it, he relives it with the background of having thought it through first.

Emergence of Self-Identify via Resolution of Fingernail Biting: The Double Bind: A "Decent-Sized" Fingernail to Chomp on

Q: Dr. Erickson has such a fantastic treatment for nail biting and thumb sucking that I just hate to mention it in front of the Master, so I asked him if he would discuss nail biting and thumb sucking, and he very kindly consented to do so.

A: A 26-year-old man with a Master's Degree in psychology walked into my office and said:

"My father took a course in hypnosis from you, and he has sent me to you now to have you cure me of fingernail biting. I have bitten my fingernails since the age of 4. And I know why. When I was 4 years old my parents decided to make me into a pianist, and they made me practice playing the piano four hours a day. I figured out that if I bit my fingernails down to the quick so that they bled my mother would take pity on me. She didn't.

"That made me really mad and I bit my fingernails some more, but she continued to make me practice the piano four hours a day. It didn't do any good, but I kept on biting my fingernails to get even with her.

"My father agreed to finance my college education as long as I practiced the piano for four hours a day. Then my father decided that I should go to medical school, and I had to flunk out four successive years because I didn't want to be a doctor. In order to keep out of medical school the last time I cheated so that every medical school in the country blacklisted me!

"Now my father wants you to hypnotize me into not biting my fingernails, but I have the habit so thoroughly established that I don't think anything can stop it; and I don't think you can hypnotize me, but I am here anyway."

"Yes," I answered, "I see that you are here. As for hypnotizing you, how much hypnosis do you really need to listen to me? I don't think you need very much, but I don't think you really like those stubby fingernails of yours either. And you have been biting them since you were 4 years old, and you are 26 years old now, and I feel rather sorry for you, because for 22 years you have been biting your fingernails and you have never gotten anything more out of it than a teensy, teensy little piece of fingernail; and you have never had a decent-sized piece of fingernail to chomp on. Twenty-two years of frustration!

"Now what I am going to suggest to you is this: You have ten fingers. Certainly you can spare one on which to grow a decent-sized fingernail, and after you have grown a decent-sized fingernail on it, bite it off, and have something worth chewing on."

The man looked at me, burst into laughter, and said, "I see exactly what you are doing, but I'll be darned, I'm going to do what you say!"

Later he explained his experience: "I decided I had nine fingernails to nibble on, and here is the finger I am really going to grow something on. But the first thing I knew, I could spare two fingers to grow decent-sized nails on—and that still left me with eight to bite. The next thing I knew, I was thinking I could get along on seven, and grow three. Well, why not four, and I would still have six. Then, what is the difference between five and six?" And he finally decided he could do all of his nibbling on one little finger, and have nine good fingernails. He was as much amused by the process as I was, and very promptly (within six months) he had ten good fingernails.

There were further results from my patient's accomplishment. His father once again insisted that he go to medical school even if he had to go abroad (having been blacklisted in all American schools). My patient discussed his intolerance of his father and his hostility toward his mother, and so on. Then he said: "I have ten good fingernails now, and I think I ought to revise my thinking on a lot of things. I am interested in law. I think I will go to law school. My father can shout and rave, he can raise Cain if he likes, but I am going to law school." He proceeded to do exactly that, and he did it very successfully.

260

Transference of Self-Identify via Example: The "Ripple Effect" in Therapy

My patient's father also had been at sword's points with another son because that son had been dating a Catholic girl, and the son gave up dating that Catholic girl. My patient dated various girls, and he happened to encounter a Catholic girl that appealed to him very much.

"You know," he explained, "I am going to marry that girl, not to spite my father, but I am going to marry her because she will make a very nice wife, and I am in love with her and she is in love with me. And maybe if I set an example my brother will change his attitude. Father has tried to make a minister out of him for years. He went and got himself engaged to a Jewish girl, meanwhile studying to be a Presbyterian minister, eventually ending up an alcoholic. When my brother finds out that I have married a Catholic girl, maybe he will realize that he has got some freedom, too."

So my patient married the Catholic girl. His father's hair curled, his mother's hair turned white—but he married the Catholic girl very happily. (I attended the wedding.)

His brother thought all this over, and said: "Well, maybe it is time I also got straightened out. There is no reason why I should drink; there is no reason why I should keep on dating this Jewish girl. She is fine, but I really don't love her, and I think I'll break off the engagement. And as for becoming a minister—I don't want to be a minister! I am going to go into the automobile business, and I am going to become a dealer in automobiles." And that is exactly what he did, after which he fell in love with a girl of his own religious faith, and he is now happily married.

Since then I have had many discussions with my lawyer patient about his marital adjustments and his family adjustments and what I did to him. He said: "I never thought that you could hypnotize me, but when I think about my experiences in your office—you never tried to hypnotize me, you never used any hypnotic technique. I have seen my father use hypnosis in his practice of medicine. You never made a gesture, you never said a word suggestive of hypnosis, but when I think about it, something did happen. When I first entered your office I could see the entire room. Within a few minutes I saw and heard only you; I didn't see the bookcases, or the filing cabinets, or the desk; I didn't know if anyone came in or not; I was just attending to what you had to say. You never discussed my conflicts with my parents, and yet those conflicts vanished very nicely."

What had I done? I knew I had a 26-year-old man who was really prepared to give me a battle. I certainly didn't want to enter a contest with him, but I did want to hold his attention, and I did want to communicate ideas to him, and I did want to communicate those ideas in a way that he could accept.

Resolution of Thumb Sucking via Division and the Double Bind: Equal Opportunity for All—Fingers!

I can think of the small child who sucked his thumb in a rather vicious way. It was his left thumb, and he would put it behind his upper incisors and pull as he sucked. The boy's father was a physician and his mother was a nurse, and they had both told that six-year-old all about the horrible things he was doing to himself by sucking his thumb—all about the kind of buck teeth he would have and how badly his face would look. They really had laid it on thick! In desperation one evening, the father phoned me and asked me to make a house call. When I arrived, Jimmy walked in sucking his thumb and pulling away at his teeth while he sucked.

"Jimmy," I said, "your father and mother have asked me to take care of you because you suck your thumb. That means that you are my patient. Do you know what it means to be somebody's patient? It means that no other doctor can open his mouth about it. And now that you are my patient your father's mouth is shut, and he can't say anything to me about what I say to you; and a nurse doesn't talk back to a doctor, and your mother is a nurse, and since you are my patient, she can't talk back to me either. You are just my patient.

"Now, let us get one thing straight. That left thumb of yours is your thumb; that mouth of yours is your mouth; those front teeth of yours are your front teeth. I think you are entitled to do anything you want to with your thumb, with your mouth, and with your teeth. They are yours, and let us get that straight. I want you to do anything you want to do."

Jimmy looked awfully surprised. He looked at his father and then he looked at his mother. He could see the dumbfounded expressions on their faces.

Then I turned to his father, asking, "Have you got anything to say?"

He said, "No, I have nothing to say."

I asked the mother and she said, "No, I have nothing to say."

Jimmy looked surprised and pleased.

"I have a little more to say to you, Jimmy," I continued. "One of the first things you learned when you went to nursery school was to take turns. You took turns with this little girl and with that little boy in doing things in nursery school. You learned to take turns in the first grade. In fact, you learned to take turns at home. When Mother serves the food she serves it first to one brother, and then it may be your turn, then it may be sister's turn, then it is Mother's turn. We always do things by turns. But I don't think you are being right or fair or good in always sucking your left thumb and never giving your right thumb a turn."

Jimmy took a deep breath as he thought over that point. He really ought to give his right thumb a turn.

"Your left thumb has received all of the sucking," I continued. "The right thumb hasn't had a turn; the first finger hasn't had a turn; not a single other finger has had a turn. Now I think you are a good little boy, and I don't think you are doing this on purpose. I think you really would like to give each of your fingers a proper turn."

Can you imagine giving a turn to ten separate digits? Can you imagine a more laborious task in the world? And Jimmy strove manfully to give his fingers (his digits) an equal turn at sucking.

Next I pointed out: "You know, Jimmy, you are over six years old now, and soon you will be a big boy of seven; and you know I have never seen a big boy or a big man that ever sucked his thumb, so you had better do all of your sucking before you are a big boy of seven." Jimmy stopped sucking his thumb before he was seven. He was a big boy then!

Resolution of Adult Bed Wetting via Structured Inconvenience: The Forty-Block Walk

The idea is to make a laborious task out of whatever the habit is—you turn a vicious habit into an awful inconvenience which the patient is very willing to give up.

I can think of the 29-year-old bed wetter who came to me and told me that he had wet the bed every night for 29 years. He was sick and tired of it. He had to live in a separate house (the guest house behind his parents' house); he couldn't go on vacation; he didn't dare go away to college; he couldn't sleep over night in a hotel; he couldn't visit relatives who lived out of town—all because he wet his bed. He wanted to know if I could do something about it. I told him, "Yes, I can, but I don't think you will like it. But you can listen to me anyway." I held his attention, and I told him what I could do about it, and he said, "Uh-huh." About three months later he came to me and said: "What was that you were going to do about my bed wetting? I think I want you to do it now."

"In taking your history," I began, "I found out that you hate to walk, even as far as across the street; that you will back your car out of the garage in order to cross the street; that you will drive to the corner in order to mail a letter; that you go to work a half hour early in order to get the parking place nearest to the entrance to where you work. In short, you are entirely dependent upon your car and you hate walking. So this is the idea.

"You wet the bed every night somewhere between midnight and one o'clock. It is your habit to awaken, change the linen on the bed, and go back to sleep in a dry bed for the rest of the night. You stack up the soiled linen after you remove it, you wash it when you come home from work, hang it up, go to bed. At midnight you stack up the wet linen, make up your bed afresh, and sleep the rest of the night. Now, I think what you ought to do is this: For the next three weeks you get an alarm

264

clock and set it for midnight, or for half past twelve, or for one o'clock—it doesn't make a bit of difference to me. When the alarm rings, you wake up, and regardless of whether your bed is wet or dry, you dress fully and you take a walk of 40 blocks— and you do that every night for three weeks. At the end of three weeks you can take a week's vacation, but the next time you find a wet bed you have another three weeks' sentence to serve by walking 40 blocks in the middle of the night."

My patient served his sentence. He hasn't dared to wet the bed since that first three weeks of night walking, because he really doesn't like walking. That is what I mean when I say that you have to make a habit inconvenient for the patient. This 29-year-old man was desperate. But since his dry bed he has joined a church; he has gone on vacations; he has traveled all through the West; he has traveled throughout the Northwest; he has traveled through the East; he has stayed in hotels; he has visited relatives in distant cities; he is dating girls and having a very delightful time. A dry bed changed his life pattern completely.

How much hypnosis did I use? Can you imagine where his attention was when I described the treatment of walking 40 blocks in the middle of the night, every night, for three long weeks? He wasn't thinking of anything except what I was saying, and he felt exceedingly compelled to do exactly what I said, because I seemed to be so absolutely, completely confident that he would be cured of his bed wetting.

Analysis and Summary: Three Cases of Symptom Resolution

So with bed wetting, with thumb sucking, or with fingernail biting, you size up the situation and then you set your goal. You see to it that the patient somehow discovers that there are a number of other things that he would rather be doing, and you make it awfully easy for him to discontinue the particular habit. That man with the Master's Degree in psychology was so amused at the proposition that he get a decent-size piece of fingernail to chomp on—awfully amused, but nevertheless his unconscious mind was listening and it recognized that I was giving him an out whereby he could set his own goal to get over his own bad habit, and he could take all the credit himself. I only asked for one fingernail. It was he who grew the rest of his fingernails; it was he who decided to give up the little fingernail. In other words, he took the entire credit. Why shouldn't he? Why do I need the credit?

Q: [Question lost in the recording.]

A: I don't really think you would call [the fingernail case] a transfer cure because the patient was doing a lot of thinking within his own mind. He could see the opportunity that I was setting up for him unconsciously; that he, himself, could take charge of a situation that he had considered impossible for years. He also recognized that I wasn't going to be a stubborn "Papa," but that I was going to be a good friend and an amusing friend.

Now in the bed wetting case, the patient's father and mother had beaten him thoroughly throughout his childhood for wetting the bed. Then I also punished him, but I punished him in a very healthy way, and it was a limited punishment. And he could work out his own, very much desired, goal. He would only have to serve that sentence for three short weeks.

Q: How did you find out about his dislike for walking?

A: In taking his history I wanted to know how he went to work and what he thought about on the way to work. I discovered that he hated cats very much, and that he always dreaded walking out to the garage in the morning to go to work. I wondered to myself why he should hate walking out to the garage—he was an able-bodied man. So I asked a few more questions: How far away is the mailbox? Do you ever mail any letters? What do you do when you mail a letter? Get in the car and drive up to the mailbox? And you say the mailbox is down at the end of the block? How far down the block is your home? It was half way down the block. He would walk out to the garage, get into the car, and drive down to the mailbox. I got my information and he knew I had that information; therefore, giving him a sentence of walking 40 blocks was not a mysterious solution. I don't know why I picked 40, but it is a good number.

Treating Examination Panics: Chance Versus Planned Feedback

[Apparently Erickson now interacts with an audience member. Material lost in the recording.]

I took advantage of Von to make a wisecrack about the examination panic, but he did something there that I learned not to do a long time ago. Whenever I take care of students' examination panics, I so govern and guide my discussion that they never have an opportunity to ask me, "Shall I call you up and tell you the results?" I don't want them to call me up. I don't want them to let me know the results, because if they feel a need to let me know the results, it is usually a need to let me know *if* they succeeded. Therefore, I see to it that they never have a chance to let me know *if* they succeeded, but I usually find out the results in some way two or three months later.

I found out the results of one student in a particularly pleasing way. This student was studying law, and he had flunked his exams five times before we worked together. A year or so after our sessions his wife came in, pregnant, and said: "After Joe passed the State Board Examination, we moved to Arizona for his practice and decided that we could start a family. Now I am going to deliver within the next two weeks. Will you handle me the way you handled Joe?"

She is pregnant again. I told her then that she really ought to come in sooner before her delivery—to give me a little more time. So with this pregnancy she came in a month early, but she still contends she had a perfectly delightful time with her first delivery.

Treating Obesity by Confronting It

Then there is the treatment of obesity. A college girl came to see me who was very, very overweight—about 100 pounds overweight. She described how she was just a "fat slob" with a very expressive face. And there was no doubt about that disagreeable expression on her face and the unhappy tones in her voice; and there was no doubt about all that misery that she must have been experiencing, emotionally. Now I don't like to give people unpleasant ideas, unpleasant feelings so I merely recognized that here was a situation in which I couldn't give her anything unpleasant—she already had it!

"I really don't think you know how unpleasant your fatness is to you," I began, "so tonight when you go to bed, first get in the nude and stand in front of a full-length mirror and really see how much you dislike all that fat you have. And if you think hard enough and look through that layer of blubber that you've got wrapped around you, you will see a very pretty feminine figure, but it is buried rather deeply. And what do you think you ought to do to get that figure excavated?" Well, she is excavating it at the rate of about five pounds a week.

It really isn't important for me to specify when I am using hypnosis and it isn't necessary for me to specify when I'm not using hypnosis. I am not going to tell you when I am using a polysyllabic word and when I am using a two-syllable word. It isn't necessary, just as long as you understand me. I simply shifted her understanding [to focus her disliking into productive channels].

Practical Suggestions for Highway Hypnosis: Paradoxical Intention, Fixation of Attention, and Physical Exercise

I amost went to sleep while driving my car on a long trip from Massachusetts to Wisconsin. When I realized I was dozing off I pulled off to the side of the road and started thinking about what the consequences could have been and about what one ought to do in this type of situation. Then I thought of what some of my patients had said about insomnia and I thought about what I had said to them about insomnia. I realized that there are two ways of handling this matter of dozing at the wheel. One way is to drive off to the side of the road, stop the car, and do your level best to go to sleep, right then

268

and there. What happens? You get wider and wider and wider awake because of your desperate effort to go to sleep—which is the exact process the insomniac goes through every night. You simply remain wide awake. Then I thought, well, there is another way of waking yourself up. When you feel awfully tired and awfully sleepy, why not get out of the car and do a little exercise—alter the circulation of your blood, do a few leg squats or a couple of push-ups—anything to bring about a change in the circulation of your blood. As a result of these changes in the circulation of your blood you are going to feel better all over, and you are going to feel wide awake.

Then when you get back in the car there are so many things you can bear in mind: now that white line in the middle of the road is a nice line to watch, but how many breaks in it can you find?; and what about watching the shoulder of the road and noting that there is a rock here, a broken post there, a shrub somewhere else. If those striped, roadside markers are regularly spaced they become as monotonous as can be—and can even produce a kind of highway hypnosis; but if you watch for something random and unexpected—a rock, a log, a shrub, a twisted stick—then you are going to stay wide awake, and in a rather easy manner.

So when you become fatigued behind the wheel, change the circulation of your blood or change your mental attitude. Once you are aware of the situation you can look about for some measure of keeping yourself awake while you continue your drive.

Parent Management by Children

I would like to give you a brief narration of parent management by children. I was sitting in a Chicago airport one morning around two o'clock when a harried mother came in with her two-year-old daughter (as closely as I could judge from the child's behavior). The mother went over to the counter and purchased a newspaper, and I observed the child look at a stuffed animal in a lower counter. The mother walked hastily away, and the child was looking over her shoulder at that stuffed animal. Mother sat down on a bench where the child had a good view of that stuffed animal. And the child looked at the toy, looked at mother, got up from the bench, and ran back and forth. Mother said, "Please sit down." The child sat down for about two seconds, then got up and ran back and forth. Mother said, "Please sit down." This kept up until the mother finally tried to hold the child down, but the little girl squirmed thoroughly. Mother said, "Lie down," and the child did, but she was very shortly up, off the bench, down on the floor, and running out. Mother jumped up and grabbed the child. The child sat down very meekly, but suddenly darted out again. The mother said, "If you want some exercise—all right!" So the child reached up and took her mother's hand and led her clear around to the counter. Mother saw the stuffed animal and said, "Maybe this will keep you quiet."

A Double Bind to Bypass a Three-Generation Identification: Death at 22 versus Rightful Payment of Bills

Let's discuss the matter of identification. A patient came in to see me very much concerned about her future. She stated that her great-grandmother had died at the age of 22 of heart disease; that her grandmother had died at the age of 22 of heart disease; that her mother had died at age 22 of heart disease; and that she herself had been diagnosed as having a cardiac condition. Her father was living, her husband was living. I interviewed both of them. The father confirmed the information about the great-grandmother, the grandmother, and the mother. The husband said that he had known about all the deaths. My patient was expecting her 22nd birthday in two months, so the question was, What should I do about it?

I asked my patient what preparation she was making for her death. (I had received a lead from her husband that legitimized such a question.) She answered that she was seeing to it that all of her bills were paid—every one of them; that she certainly wasn't going to die until every last bill was paid. Next I asked her if she were familiar with the practice of various companies, of various business people: some like to be paid on the first of the month; some like to be paid on the 15th of the month; some like to be paid at the end of the month.

I then raised the question of whether or not companies and businesses had the right to set the date of payment. And I went into that issue at considerable length, and I led her way out on a limb in which she agreed that anyone who rendered services or goods of any sort had the right to set the date of payment. As I looked at my calendar, I told her that I expected payment for the present office call exactly fourteen months from today. She came in fourteen months later and paid her bill, because I had also pointed out: "You know, if your grandmother, your great-grandmother, your mother had lived to be 23, they probably would have lived a lot longer." And she agreed in the trance state that they probably would have. She couldn't die until she paid my bill, and she couldn't die after the age of 23 until sufficient time had passed. I simply put her in a bind very effectively, but she didn't know that I was putting her in a bind at the time. My narration about rightful date of payment seemed so useless and needless, but the point is to draw patients out on a limb and get an idea across to them.

Countertransference in Medical Students: Developing a Respectful Attitude toward All Patients

Now here is an important question: In your endeavor to analyze and control the attitudes of patients, how do you subdue your own countertransference so that anxiety is therefore not aroused?

I have often taken my medical students through cancer clinics because I think they ought to see terminal cases of cancer; I think they ought to see all the ulcerations and all the very difficult things that result from neglectful cases. This was in the County Hospital in Detroit, Michigan, and my medical students were rather repulsed by the appearance of the patients' wounds and by their generally depressing condition. After my students were thoroughly repulsed and had manifested thoroughly their adverse reactions, I pointed out:

"You are reacting adversely to those patients. Why? Aren't they the patients that are affording you a medical education? How do you expect to make your living except by meeting your patients, by respecting and liking them—by thoroughly liking them. Those patients allow this County Hospital to function, and this County Hospital is giving you a good share of your medical education, and you are not paying for all of your education by any means. Don't you think you ought to be grateful to those patients? Why are you repulsed? Why are you offended by them?"

I also would take medical students through the back wards of the psychiatric section and do the same thing with them. You simply ought not to have any other attitude toward patients than one of sympathy and liking and respect. It is fine to dislike cancer; that is an impersonal dislike. You don't have to like a TB germ. I like Dave Cheek, but I don't like any TB germ, and I don't care how well dyed it is! That is what I teach my students about how they ought to feel toward their patients.

Control versus Utilization of Patient Behavior; Determining Patient Welfare; Knowing the Right Time and Place

Now, do you control patients? I don't think you do. I don't think you should even try. You ought to talk to patients; you ought to analyze their behaviors; and then you ought to wonder what you can do to help them. I try to utilize their behaviors in a helpful, constructive way, because certainly I am not qualified to control their behavior. I don't know how to tell you how to drive your car home for the simple reason that I know nothing about your reflex responses, your reaction time, or anything of that sort; I am simply not qualified to tell you how to drive a car, even though I myself know how to drive a car. I do not know how you react to red lights or green lights, or how you react to pedestrians; so the best that I could do would be to give you a whole set of instructions that would fit *my* driving behavior. It certainly would not fit your driving behavior, because my driving behavior might be too rapid or too slow, too aggressive or too passive. I just don't know how it would differ from yours.

You don't control another person's behavior. You recognize it, you aid patients in utilizing it, you aid patients in directing it to meet their needs; but you do not work with patients to achieve your own goals. The goal is their welfare, and if you succeed in bringing about their welfare you are indirectly affecting your own welfare.

How do we decide what is for the patient's welfare? When you get to know your patient well enough you can recognize that there are certain things in general that he should not do. Really, he should not get drunk every weekend, without fail. That is not good for him. You can ask him and he will tell you so, too. He ought not to be wasting his money gambling. He will tell you that is so, too. There are certain general things, and as you talk to your patient you can discover what his standards of living really are. Now his standards of living may not be the same as my standards of living, but each person is entitled to his own standards, and I haven't got the right to force my standards, whether lower or higher, on any patient.

QUESTIONS AND ANSWERS

Q: [Isn't the self-destructive adult still reacting to] a parent who said, essentially, "You will never amount to anything—you are no damn good?" So the adult feels that by gambling, or biting his fingernails, or smoking four packages of cigarettes a day, or drinking every weekend, that he is really doing what was intended for his welfare. Wouldn't he feel that, perhaps, you weren't being kind to him if you tried to change his pattern?

A: My statement to such a patient would be: "Your dad feels that you should be a very, very clever second-storey workman; that you ought to be able to sneak up to a second storey and rob the bedrooms therein, and do a perfectly beautiful job of it. Your dad says that. His friends say that. What do you really think about it?''

Q: But suppose the patient doesn't even remember what his father said, and just comes to you for help with his alcoholism?

A: If he comes to me and says, "I think it is all right to drink and to get drunk," I am going to agree with him. Under what circumstances do you drink? There are certain circumstances where you do certain things. I think it is a very desirable thing to brush your teeth, but please don't do it at the table. There is nothing criminal about it, there is nothing really wrong with it, but don't do it at the table. If you want to get drunk, do it in the right place, in the right company, and to the right degree. And then you ask the patient to analyze his behavior and to better understand it.

Q: Perhaps there was another misunderstanding when I asked where *you* learned psychiatry, and you were explaining how you studied the methods of getting attention and getting a teacher to do this or that. I came upon a sudden realization: This was Erickson's way of learning how to teach, of learning how to get a person to see something clearly and to do something about it. It was not, as it may have sounded to some members of the audience, a manipulation—any more than it is manipulative for the coach to ask an athlete who thinks he is no good and can't win that hurdle race to go over those hurdles ten times or twenty times in order to build up his strength and his ability. You are the coach, and you are learning to coach to the best of your ability.

A: That is right, and you observe behavior so that you have a better understanding of it, and then when you see good behavior in somebody you encourage it; when you see bad behavior you let the person understand that he is competent to behave better than that, to give a better performance.

Practical Application of the Fractional Approach to Behavior Utilization: The Champion Shot-Putter

I can think of Dallas Long who used to be the champion shot putter at 67 feet and 10 inches. The world's record had been 61 feet and a few inches for years and years, but Dallas changed that. Then Matson came along and made it 70 feet and 7 inches.

[Dallas came to me for help long before he was champion of anything.] I explained to him: "You are a great big boy; you weigh 250 pounds; you are 6 feet 6 inches tall; and, you know, I think it is absurd for you to believe that you can't hurl that shotput any further than 58 feet. I think that is awfully wrong. I don't know how far you can put that shot, but I do know that men who are smaller than you, who are not as strong as you, who weigh less than you have put it more than 58 feet. Now, won't you tell me the difference between 58 feet, and 58 feet and 1/100th of an inch? Do you think you could put the ball, the shotput, 1/100th of an inch further?

Dallas said, "Yes," and then he went out and set a national high school record, and then he went out and set other national records, and then he went on to first place in the Olympics. Later he set the world record, only to be beaten by Matson. But Dallas had sat in my office after his world record, and we had agreed that sooner or later Dallas ought to look forward to seeing somebody beat his record, and I expect Dallas was as pleased as I was when his record was beaten. Why shouldn't Dallas be pleased at human accomplishment? And I think that is the way one ought to treat human behavior.

Patient Hypnotizability: Complex Relations between Conscious and Unconscious

Q: What are the personality traits and other factors that you look for as indications of hypnotizability when you first see a patient?

A: I really do not know what the traits are. They all add up

275

to a different sum. Each individual is an individual. You recognize the individuality of that person and you try to respond to that person as an individual. You can recognize that this person, because of your accumulated experience, will enter hypnosis slowly, and that one will go into hypnosis readily, and that one you had better delay a day or so, or a week or so, maybe a month or so.

Take the example of, say, neurodermatitis. I understand that the cause of this condition is at the unconscious level. If the unconscious is so smart, smart enough to know how much of the condition to let go of as determined under hypnosis, why does it not let go of it spontaneously? This seems paradoxical. The conscious mind must also have something to do with it. How often have you done something awfully foolish and awfully stupid in full conscious awareness, and then wished like anything that you hadn't done it? You knew better at the time, and you feel so disgusted with yourself for doing it, because you did know better than to lose your temper with so-and-so; you did know better than to cuss out that traffic cop; you did know better than to start an argument with your mother-in-law. And you get so disgusted with yourself. That is at the conscious level, too; and you know it consciously, and you get disgusted at the conscious level.

But does it ever occur to you that you can do something quite innocently on a conscious level and your unconscious, out of its great wealth of wisdom, says: "Look here, that is the wrong sort of thing to do. Now do it differently!"? Yet you consciously insist on doing it the wrong way. How many times has that obese woman looked at that great big cake and said, "I'll just take a little piece," knowing consciously at the time that she is lying to herself—that she is going to take one dozen little pieces. She has lied to herself, and her unconscious gets so disgusted and says: "All right, if you want to make a pig of yourself, eat the rest of it"; and the unconscious tends to punish the conscious. Now when you get the unconscious mind interested in helping out the stupid conscious mind then you can get the unconscious to recognize that there is a certain amount of the difficulty that can be relinquished. Sometimes I

276

have had to explain this idea to patients in the deep trance, and they have listened attentively and then they agree, "Well, yes, it is my unconscious punishing my conscious mind, and that is why I have this neurotic tendency."

Catatonia versus Catalepsy: A Matter of Relationship

Q: How do you compare the catatonia of the psychotic patient with the catalepsy of the hypnotic subject?

A: If you examine the catalepsy that the catatonic schizophrenic manifests, you will discover that it is in relationship to the patient himself. His catalepsy belongs to him, and you are not going to control it; you are not going to direct it. You can lift his arm and he will leave it where you have lifted it, but he has lost all sense of reality; his arm, so far as he is concerned, may be there or it may be here, but the arm position belongs entirely to him.

When you lift the arm in hypnosis, however, the subject knows where you have put his arm unless, of course, you specifically ask him to forget it. But the hypnotic subject is aware of the arm position and experiences it as a part of the relationship between you and him. In schizophrenia there is no relationship between you and the patient, and so if you want to pick up that thing he has rejected, well, that is your business; and the patient will leave that thing that you picked up wherever you leave it, but his identity remains something entirely internal to him.

BIBLIOGRAPHY

Asbaugh, D. *Nevada's Turbulent Yesterday.* Los Angeles: West-ernlore, 1963.

Bandler, R., & Grinder, J. *The Patterns of the Hypnotic Tech-niques of Milton H. Erickson, M.D.* Vol. I. Palo Alto, Calif.: Science & Behavior Books, 1975.

Bateson, G., Jackson, D., Haley, J., & Weakland, J. Toward a Theory of Schizophrenia. *Behavioral Science,* 1956, *1,* 251-264.

Beahrs, J. Integrating Erickson's Approach. *The American Jour-nal of Clinical Hypnosis,* 1977, *20,* 55-68.

Beahrs, J. *That Which Is: An Inquiry into the Nature of Energy, Ethics, and Mental Health.* Palo Alto, Calif.: Science & Be-havior Books, 1977.

Bergantino, L. *Psychotherapy, Insight and Style: The Existen-tial Moment.* Boston: Allyn & Bacon, 1981.

Brain/Mind Bulletin. Hypnotist Describes Natural Rhythm of Trance Readiness. *Brain/Mind Bulletin, 6,* March, 1981.

Bucke, M. A. *Cosmic Consciousness.* New York: Innes & Son, 1901. Republished by Dutton, 1967.

Cheek, D. Unconscious Perceptions of Meaningful Sounds Dur-ing Surgical Anesthesia as Revealed Under Hypnosis. *The American Journal of Clinical Hypnosis,* 1959, *1,* 103-113.

Cooper, L., & Erickson, M. H. *Time Distortion in Hypnosis.* Baltimore: Williams & Wilkins, 1954.

Cooper, L., & Erickson, M. H. *Time Distortion in Hypnosis.* (2nd ed.) Baltimore: Williams & Wilkins, 1959.

Erickson, M. H. *Advanced Techniques of Hypnosis and Therapy: Selected Papers of Milton H. Erickson, M.D.* Edited by Jay Haley. New York: Grune & Stratton, 1967.

Erickson, M. H. A Special Inquiry with Aldous Huxley into the Nature and Character of Various States of Consciousness. *The Collected Papers of Milton H. Erickson on Hypnosis.* Edited by Ernest L. Rossi. Vol. I. The Nature of Hypnosis and Suggestion. New York: Irvington, 1980.

Erickson, M. H. *A Teaching Seminar of Milton H. Erickson.* Edited by Jeffrey Zeig. New York: Brunner-Mazel, 1980.

Erickson, M. H. Further Experimental Investigation of Hypnosis: Hypnotic and Nonhypnotic Realities. *The Collected Papers of Milton H. Erickson on Hypnosis.* Edited by Ernest L. Rossi. Vol. I. The Nature of Hypnosis and Suggestion. New York: Irvington, 1980.

Erickson, M. H. Initial Experiments Investigating the Nature of Hypnosis. *The Collected Papers of Milton H. Erickson on Hypnosis.* Edited by Ernest L. Rossi. Vol. I. The Nature of Hypnosis and Suggestion. New York: Irvington, 1980.

Erickson, M. H. Pantomime Techniques in Hypnosis and the Implications. *The Collected Papers of Milton H. Erickson on Hypnosis.* Edited by Ernest L. Rossi. Vol. I. The Nature of Hypnosis and Suggestion. New York: Irvington, 1980.

Erickson, M. H. Pediatric Hypnotherapy. *The Collected Papers of Milton H. Erickson on Hypnosis.* Edited by Ernest L. Rossi. Vol. IV. Innovative Hypnotherapy. New York: Irvington, 1980.

Erickson, M. H. Possible Detrimental Effects from Experimental Hypnosis. *The Collected Papers of Milton H. Erickson on Hypnosis.* Edited by Ernest L. Rossi. Vol. I. The Nature of Hypnosis and Suggestion. New York: Irvington, 1980.

Erickson, M. H. *The Collected Papers of Milton H. Erickson on Hypnosis.* (4 vols.) Edited by Ernest L. Rossi. New York: Irvington, 1980.

Erickson, M. H., Haley, J., & Weakland, J. A Transcript of a Trance Induction. *The Collected Papers of Milton H. Erickson on Hypnosis.* Edited by Ernest L. Rossi. Vol. I. The Nature of Hypnosis and Suggestion. New York: Irvington, 1980.

Erickson, M. H., Hershman, S., & Secter, I. *The Practical Application of Medical and Dental Hypnosis.* New York: Julian Press, 1961.

Erickson, M. H., & Rossi, E. L. *Hypnotherapy: An Exploratory Casebook.* New York: Irvington, 1979.

Erickson, M. H., & Rossi, E. L. Autohypnotic Experiences of Milton H. Erickson. *The Collected Papers of Milton H. Erickson on Hypnosis.* Edited by Ernest L. Rossi. Vol. I. The Nature of Hypnosis and Suggestion. New York: Irvington, 1980.

Erickson, M. H., & Rossi, E. L. Varieties of Double Bind. *The Collected Papers of Milton H. Erickson on Hypnosis.* Edited by Ernest L. Rossi. Vol. I. The Nature of Hypnosis and Suggestion. New York: Irvington, 1980.

Erickson, M. H., & Rossi, E. L. *Experiencing Hypnosis: Therapeutic Approaches to Altered States.* New York: Irvington, 1981.

Erickson, M. H., Rossi, E. L., & Rossi, S. I. *Hypnotic Realities.* New York: Irvington, 1976.

Grinder, J., Delozier, J., & Bandler, R. *The Patterns of the Hypnotic Techniques of Milton H. Erickson, M.D.* Vol. 2. Palo Alto, Calif.: Science & Behavior Books, 1975.

Haley, J. *Uncommon Therapy: The Psychiatric Techniques of Milton H. Erickson.* New York: Norton, 1973.

Hiatt, J., & Kripke, D. Ultradian Rhythms in Waking Gastric Activity. *Psychosomatic Medicine,* 1975, *37,* 330-325.

Jung, C. G. *The Archetypes and the Collective Unconscious.* New York: Pantheon Books, 1959.

Ravitz, L. J. Electrometric Correlates of the Hypnotic State. *Science,* 1950, *112,* 341.

Ravitz, L. J. History, Measurement, and Applicability of Periodic Changes in the Electromagnetic Field in Health and Disease. *American Archives of New York Science,* 1962, *92,* 1144-1201.

Ravitz, L. J. Leaders in Contemporary Science. *Journal of the American Society of Psychosomatic Dentistry and Medicine,* 1981, *28,* 3-7.

Rosen, S. *My Voice Will Go With You: The Teaching Tales of Milton H. Erickson, M.D.* New York: Norton, 1982.

Rossi, E. L. *Dreams and the Growth of Personality*. New York: Pergamon, 1972.

Rossi, E. L. The Cerebral Hemispheres in Analytical Psychology. *Journal of Analytical Psychology*, 1977, *9*, 32–51.

Rossi, E. L. Psychological Shocks and Creative Moments in Psychotherapy. *The Collected Papers of Milton H. Erickson on Hypnosis*. Edited by Ernest L. Rossi. Vol. IV. Innovative Hypnotherapy. New York: Irvington, 1980.

Rossi, E. L. Hypnosis and Ultradian Cycles: A New State(s) Theory of Hypnosis? *The American Journal of Clinical Hypnosis*, 1982, *25*, 21–32.

Watzlawick, P. *The Language of Change*. New York: Basic Books, 1978.

MILTON H. ERICKSON:
A PHOTOGRAPHIC PORTFOLIO

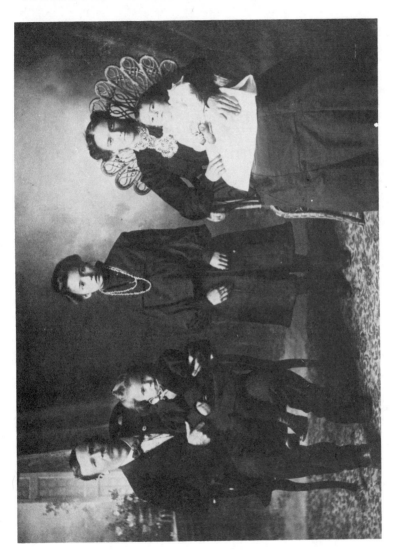

Albert Erickson, young Milton, sister Florence, Clara Erickson, and sister Winifred. 1905.

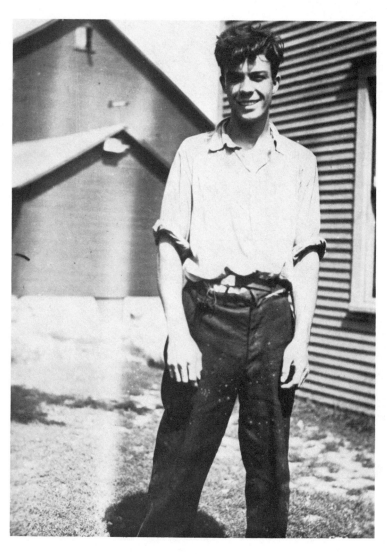

A triumphant Milton standing unaided after his first bout with polio. (Cover Photo) 1919.

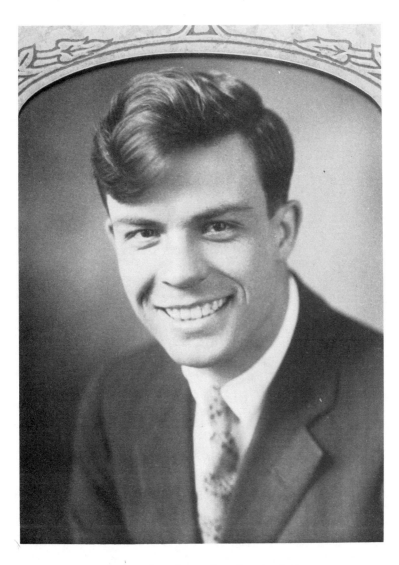

High school graduation. 1919.

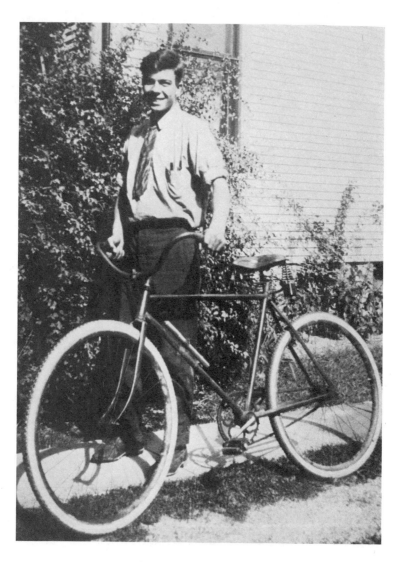

Early college days. 1922.

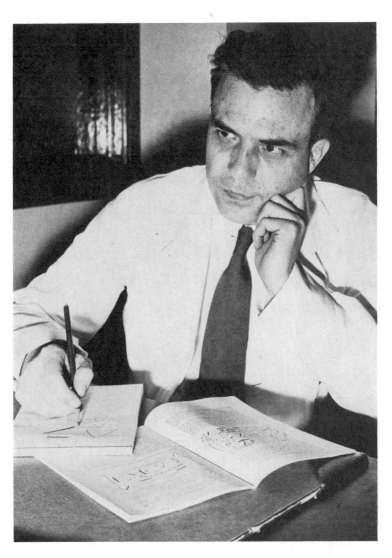

Early research years in Eloise, Michigan. 1942.

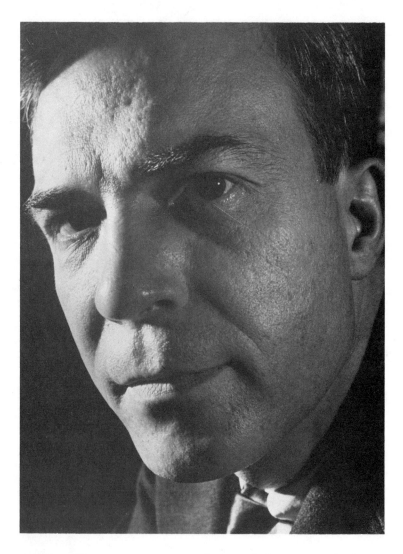

During the war years, when Erickson worked on government projects with Margaret Mead. (Photo by Jerry Cooke) 1945.

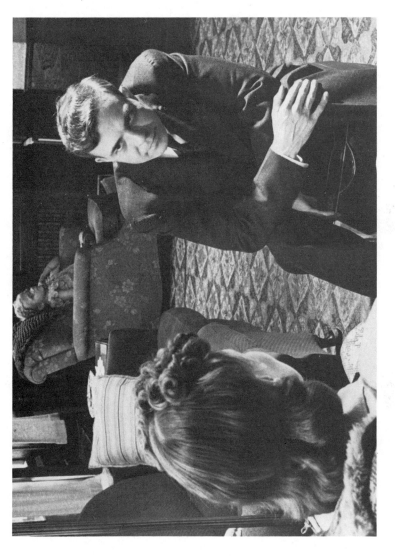

Photo taken for *American Magazine*. Elizabeth Erickson, Milton, and daughter Betty Alice in their Eloise, Michigan livingroom. (Photo by Jerry Cooke) 1945.

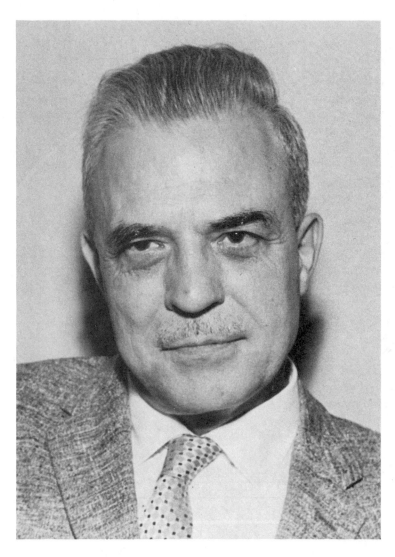

Erickson during the early years of the Los Angeles Seminars in Hypnosis, when he collaborated with Aldous Huxley in a study of altered states of consciousness. 1950.

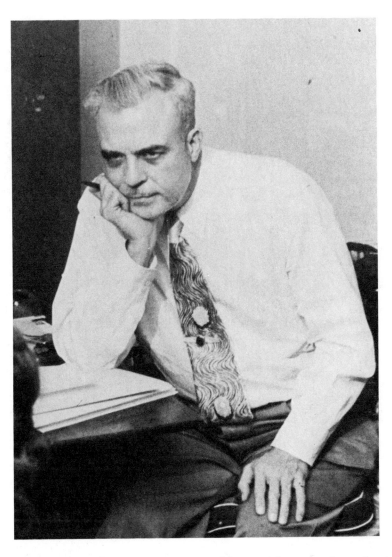

Photo taken of Erickson working with a patient for *Parade Magazine*. **The famous Erickson gaze. 1956.**

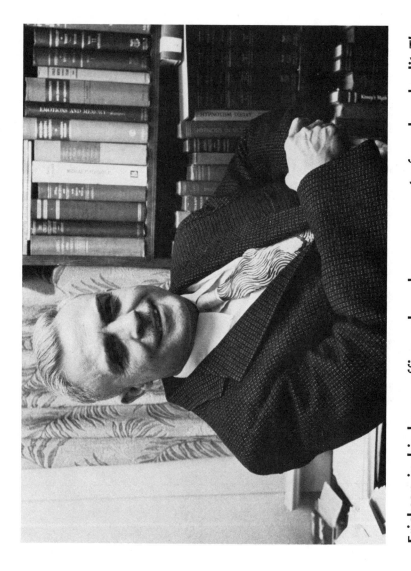

Erickson in his home office, where he was soon to found and edit *The American Journal of Clinical Hypnosis.* 1956.

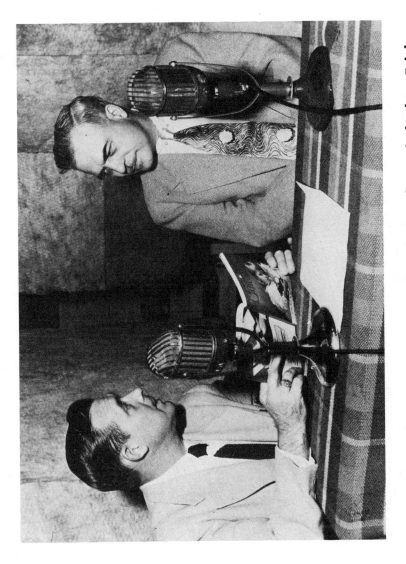

A radio interview in Washington, D.C., during the period when Erickson was a founding member of The American Society of Clinical Hypnosis. (Reni Photos) 1956.

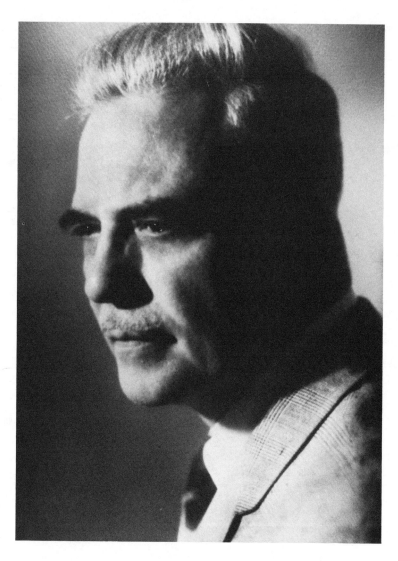

A reflective Erickson at the peak of his career. 1959.

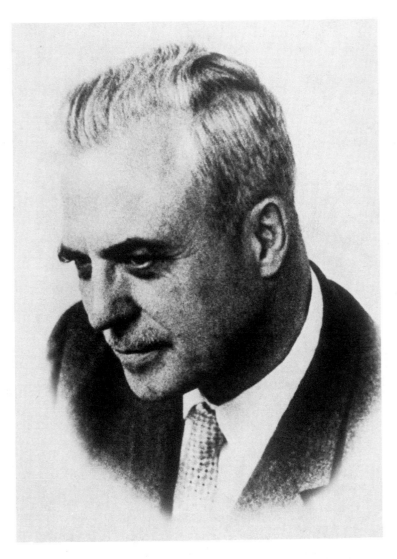

Erickson in Venezuela on one of his many international tours, where he developed his famous Pantomime Technique for inducing hypnosis without the use of language. 1960.

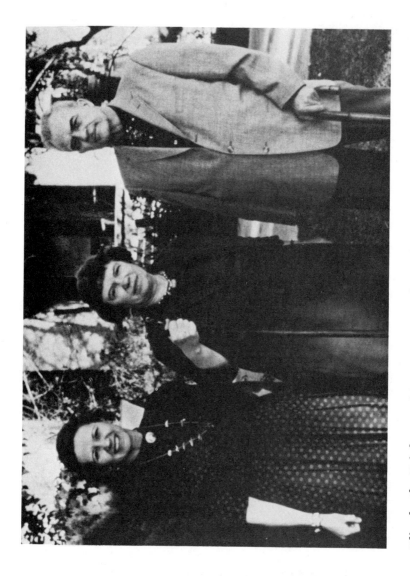

Elizabeth Erickson, Margaret Mead, and Milton during his leadership years. 1963.

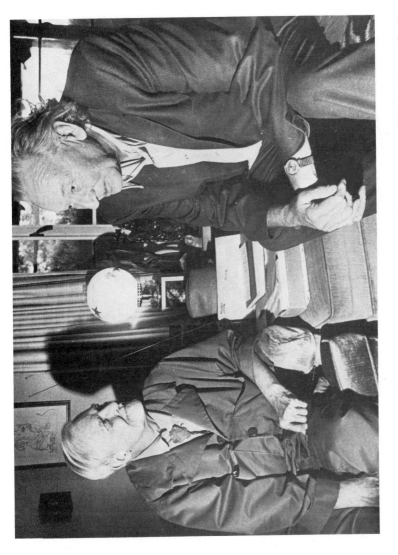

Erickson and Gregory Bateson discussing the human condition from their respective points of view. 1977.

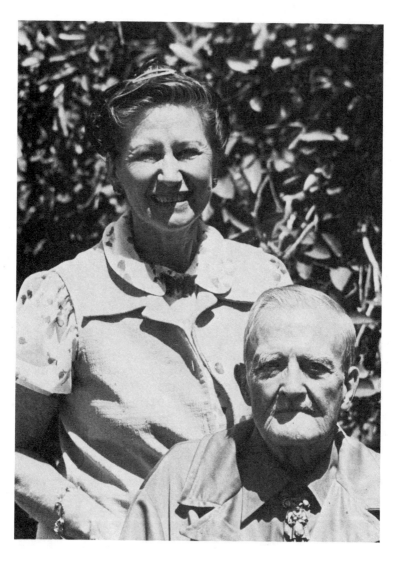

Erickson with wife, Betty, his ever-present helpmate and collaborator. (Photo by Rene Bergermaier) 1977.

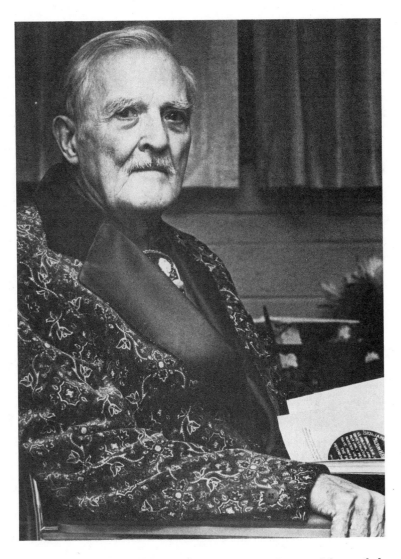

Erickson holding the Benjamin Franklin Gold Medal,
awarded to him by The International Society of Hypnosis for his outstanding contributions to the field.
1977.

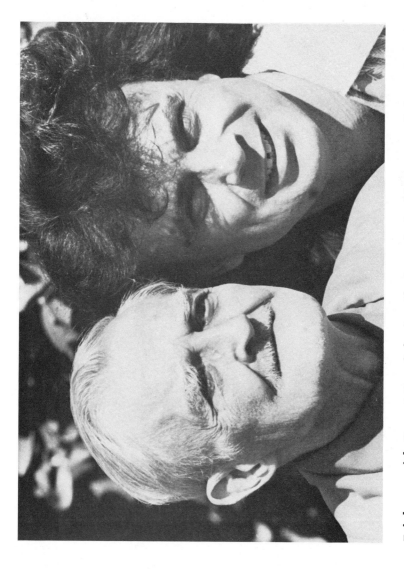

Erickson with Ernest Rossi during their period of intense collaboration on Milton's life work. (Photo by Rene Bergermaier) 1978.

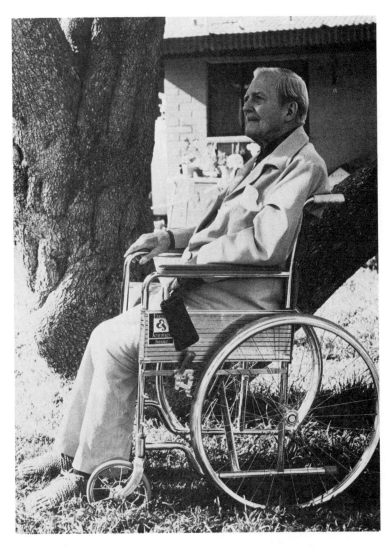

A month before his death, a quiet sage. 1980.

INDEX

Acute obsessional phobia 68
Age regression
    confusion and **254**
    visual hallucination and 255
Altered state *(See also* Conscious-
    ness, Hypnosis, Reality, Un-
    consciousness) 80, **99f**
    hypnosis as 107
    symptom relief and 129
Amnesia 71, 88
    Erickson's 17
    structured 125
    time distortion and 228
Analytical psychology 189
Anesthesia (Analgesia) *(See also*
    Pain)
    analgesia 124, 226
    confusion and 171, 234
    indirect approach for 168
Anger (Frustration)
    evoking new learning 190
Angina symptoms 214
Appetite 201
Archetypes
    collective unconscious and 188
Ashbaugh, D. 2

Assagioli, R. 47
Asthma
    fractional approach to 198
Attention
    directing 177
    fixating 70, 169, 174, 177,
    262
    focusing 90, 177
    highly focused 24
    highway hypnosis and 268
    patient behavior and 169
    talking sense and 177
    unexpected trance and 174
Authoritarian approach
    shock and 211
Autohypnosis
    conscious and unconscious in
    250f
    Erickson's 19
    Mrs. Erickson's discoveries
    250
    stages of 252

Bandler, R. 53
Bateson, G. **41f,** 57
Beahrs, J. 54

Bergantino, L. 54
Body
    awareness 123
    movement in trance 149
    trance and 91, 149
Brain damage (organic) 190
Brain functioning
    dysfunction and 187
    hypnosis and **182f**
    psychopathology and **187f**
Bucke, M. 47

Case illustrations
    acute obsessional phobia 68
    Allen's hundred stitches 142
    amnesia for pain 228
    appetite 201
    bedwetting 264
    Betty Alice's practical joke 179
    Betty Alice's vicarious learning 234
    Burt's car keys 246
    calloused pain nerves 110
    cardiac neurosis 113
    Cathy's horrible chanting 168
    champion shot-putter 275
    death at twenty-two 270
    Eva's single treatment 206
    examination panic 267
    fingernail biting 259
    floating nude men 116
    fortieth birthday phobia 68
    forty-block walk 264
    fuck-for-fun 205
    hopeless student 73
    interrupted words 188
    Janet's pease porridge hot 190
    Joe's dry bed 175
    life transformation 72
    Miss O 105

Mrs. Erickson's discoveries 250f
Mrs. Erickson's regression **256f**
Mrs. Linden's double bind 139
    obesity 267
    polysyllabic couple 203
    psychotic case 67
    rapid healing 72
    Robert's red blood 177
    Salaame Annie 208
    self-identity 259, 261
    sexual functioning 203, 206
    symptom resolution **265f**
    tall building phobia 196
    temper tantrums 105
    thumbsucking 116f, 262
    time distortion for pain 228
    traumatic scratch 115
    untutored boy 67
Catalepsy 86
    catatonia and 277
    trance and 87
Cheek, D. 80, 219
Children
    hyperactive 104
    hypnotic approach to 115
    negative suggestion with 123
    parent management 269
    psychology of 73
    two-year-old's technique 64
Communication
    hypnosis and **182f**
    ideas as **182f**
    research project 41
Conflict
    verbal and nonverbal 162
Confusion (Doubt) **79f**
    age regression and 254
    analgesia and 171
    disorientation and 234

304

Erickson's discovery of 40
pain and 234
physiological functioning and
  201
receptivity and 171
Conscious Unconscious
complex relations of 275
double bind 253
hypnotizability and 275
Consciousness
cosmic 47
higher 47
Cooper, L. 37
Corrective Emotional Experience
  151
Countertransference
medical students and 271
Creative moments
shock and 203
Cues
nonverbal 240

Dancing 23
Death
at twenty-two 270
self-induced 180
Delozier, J. 53
Demonstrations (Demonstrating)
catalepsy **86f**
confusion (doubt) 79
double bind 138
eye closure 82
hallucination 155
hand levitation 80
implication 80
Joan 86
June 138
Mary 77f
Mrs. L 138
posthypnotic suggestion 87,
  95

potentials facilitating 95
questions 79
relaxation 144
response attentiveness 87
subtle cues 154f
touch 81
trance awakening 91
trance deepening 82, 90
vocal cues 79
Dental (Dentistry) 101, 116, 140
Depotentiating
rigid beliefs 203, 206
Dissociation
anesthesia and **231f**, 234
light trance and 145
regression (two-stage) 258
tactile guidance for 147
trance awakening and 147
Distraction *(See also* Confusion)
physiological functioning and
  201f
Double bind 48, 80, 136
classic 42
conscious-unconscious 253
example of 175, 259, 262
misuse of 141
practical applications of 142
symptom relief and 136
three-generation identification
  270
time 80
trance induction 138
varieties of 9
Doubt *(See also* Confusion)
discharging **253f**
Dreams 45
Dunbar, F. 181

Eisenbeiss, J. 28
EKG 69
Electromagnetic field 48

Erickson, Albert **1f**
Erickson, Clara **1f**
Erickson, Elizabeth (Betty) 26, 35, **178f, 250f,** 257
Erickson, Milton H.
  altered perceptions **5f**
  American Society of Clinical Hypnosis **38f**
  autohypnosis **18f, 25f, 30f**
  Benjamin Franklin Gold Medal 55
  biographical sketch **1f**
  clinical director (Arizona State Hospital) 27
  colleagues, early 38
  college and medical training **14f**
  color blindness 5
  constitutional differences **5f**
  director of psychiatric research 26
  dyslexia 6
  early family history **1f**
  early life **5f**
  early papers 21
  early research years 22
  editor 38
  editorials 17
  "Eric the Badger" 15
  family man 43
  humerous stories 27
  hypnosis, self-discovery **10f**
  Japanese character structure 27
  journalistic projects 16, 27
  leadership years 36
  manipulative 40
  marriage 26
  maturing professional 27
  Nazi propaganda analysis 27
  natural man **1f**
  neurological examination 28
  pain **29f**
  personal physician 28
  polio **10f,** 28
  Sage of Phoenix 42
  self-exploration 12
  teacher (Miss Walsh) 8
  time distortion work 37
  unconscious **35f**
  U.S. Rifle Team 38
  viking spirit 2
  Wayne County General Hospital **25f**
  Worcester State Hospital **23f**
Examination panics 267
Experiential
  hypnotic induction 163
  learning **161f**
  past learning 163
Eyelid fluttering 145

Feedback
  chance vs. planned 267
Fingernail biting case 259
Fractional approach
  behavior utilization and 275
  pain and 231
  phobia reduction and 196, 198
Frazier's *The Golden Bow* 187

Gorton, B. **38f**
Grinder, J. 53

Habit problems
  awareness for 116
  bruxism 121
  gagging 118
  thumbsucking 116
  tongue habits 118
Haley, J. 40, **45f**

306

Hallucination 68, 72, 116
  age regression and 255
  questions and 153
  visual 155, 213, 255
Healing images 78
Hershman, S. **38f**
Hiatt, J. 85
Highway hypnosis 268
Hilgard, E. 42
History
  hypnosis 61
  medical 61
  psychoanalysis 63
  scientific 61
Hull, C. 19, 105
Humor 64
Huxley, A. **37f**, 57, 251
Hypnosis
  brain functioning and **182f**
  demonstration 76
  group 77
  highway 268
  history of 61f
  hyper-alert state in 70
  indirect 77, **79f**
  inner absorption and 186f
  learning and **250f**
  motivation in 68
  practice and review in 238
  purpose of **76**
  relaxation in 144
  self-examination and 186
  spontaneous 105
Hypnotic
  behavior 105, 159, 161
  dreams 45
  induction *(See also* Demonstrations, Trance) **163f**
  introspection 107
  orientation 100
  not knowing 80

realities 47
response (single) 247
self-examination 186
sensations 109
Hypnotic phenomena
  amnesia 71, 88, 125
  anesthesia (analgesia) 124
  building 83
  hand levitation 80
  inner absorption 186
  subtle cues and 154
Hypnotizability 275

Iatrogenic
  disease 221
  health 221
Illusory choice 82, 136
  covering all possibilities of
    response 175
Implication 80, 150, 151
Indirect
  anesthesia 231, 234
  hypnosis 77, 48
  ideodynamic focusing **246f**
  suggestion 64
  trance deepening 250
Insight
  MHE's view of 49
Introspection
  experiment 107
  hypnotic 107
Inward focusing
  approaches to 164
  hypnotic induction and **163f**

Jackson, D. 41
Jackson, H. C. L. 27
Jenner, E. 61
Jung, C. G. 188

Kripke, D. 85

Kroger, W. 38
Kubie, L. 57, 82

Larson, J. A. 27f
Lashley's experiments 181
Learned limitations 88
Learning *(See also* Potentials)
  neurological 217
  new **96f, 181f**
  physiological 217
  somatic 217
  vicarious 234
Life transformation, spontaneous
  72
Lustig, H. 53

McTear, professor 256
Mandy, T. 38
Manipulation
  Erickson's view of 40
Maslow, A. 47
Mead, Margaret 26, 38, 57
Memories
  in trance induction **101f**
Mental mechanisms
  Erickson's papers on 21
  power of 180
  self-induced death 180
Moore, Elizabeth (Betty) 26
Moore, M. 28
Moss, A. 38
Muscle sensation 123
Mystical 47

Naturalistic utilization techniques
  48
Neurodermatitis 203
Neuro-Linguistic Programming
  (NLP) 53
Nevada's Turbulent Yesterday 2

New
  learning 190
  potentials **182f**
  startle technique and 213
  understanding 213
Not knowing 80

Obesity 267
Obstetrics 100

Pain **217f**
  absence of 171
  amnesia and 182, 226, 228
  anesthesia and analgesia 226
  association and 220
  attributes 221
  confusion and 234
  construct 218
  control 168, 177, **217f**
  division 22
  eighty-percent loss 236
  expectation and 218
  fractional approach 236
  habit 220
  hypnotic intervention in **221f,**
    224
  itch and 173
  memories 218
  neutral sensations and 220
  pleasure and 126
  psychological frameworks 221
  reinterpretation 222
  relief 101, 137
  removal 173
  sensation substitution 227
  symptom substitution 227
  temporal considerations 218
  time distortion 228
Pantomime technique 39
Parran, T. 63

Patient framework **196f**
Pattie, F. 38
Pavlovian theory 23
Pearson, R. 132
Permissive technique
  unconscious potentials and
  165
Peters, S. 55
Phenomenological approach 45
Phobias
  fractional approach 196
  treatment of 120
Physiological functioning 199
Pillsbury, W. B. 21
Posthypnotic suggestion
  behavioral inevitabilities and
  184
  demonstrating 87, 95
Potentials
  brain functioning and 187
  facilitating **50f**, 75, 77, 79, 87,
  95f, 165f
  dysfunctions and 187
  new and lost learning 181
  untapped **182f**
Princehorn 67, 188
Pseudoscientific explanations 78
Psychiatry
  learning 245
  practical experimentation in
  245
Psychoanalysis 57, 63
Psychological shock (See also
  Shock and surprise)
  authoritarian approach 211
  openmindedness 214
Psychopathology
  aphasia and 188
  brain functions and **187f**
  correction of **198**

reverse potentials 67
untutored boy 67f
Psychosis 67, 116
  iatrogenic 70
  schizophrenia 187
Psychosomatic medicine
  hypnosis and 181
Psychosynthesis 47
Psychotherapy
  patient needs and 215
Pupil dilation 179

Questions **79f**
  dental problems and 140
  double binding 81
  opening the mind 214
  shock and **214**

Raddatz, P. (Mrs.) 3
Rapport 116, 136
Ravitz, L. J. 48, **51**
Raynaud's Disease 202
Reality
  dissection to alter 224
Reality orientation
  patients' 113, 131
  trance deepening and 131
  versus hypnotic 100
Receptivity
  confusion and 171
Reed, Dr. 78
Reframing 54
Regression
  objective understanding and
  258
  questions and 153
  two stage 258
Reiser, M. 55
Relaxation 240

Resistance
    bypassing 136
    discharging 241, 244
    utilizing **167f, 237f**
Response
    attentiveness 87, 231
    behavior and 238
    covering all possibilities 175
    demonstration 87
    hypnotic 238
    readiness 159
    subject selection and 76f
Rogers, C. 47
Rosen, H. 64
Rosen, S. 54
Rossi, E. xf, 1f, **28f, 42f**, 79f,
    85f, 97f, 189
    Erickson relationship **45f**
Ryan, M. xif

Samadhi (Nirvana) 57
Schizophrenia *(See also* Psychosis)
    toward a theory of 41
Secter, I. **38f**
Self identity 259
    transference and 261
Sexual functioning
    restoring via shock and surprise
        203, 206
Sharp, F. ixf
Shock (and surprise)
    depotentiating obsessive-
        compulsive behavior 208
    depotentiating rigid beliefs
        203, 206
    openmindedness and **213f**
    psychological shocks 46
    sexual functioning 203, 206
    startle technique and 213
    well-being and 206
Sleep 91

Soul 47
Startle technique *(See also* Shock
    and surprise) 213
Stories 78
Subtle cues
    hypnotic phenomena and 154
Suggestion
    compound 165
    contingent 184
    direct 82
    implication 80, 150f, 241
    indirect 84, 126, 153
    negative 123, 184, 241
    resistance and 241
    vocal dynamics 242
Superstition
    and hypnosis 61
Symptom(s) *(See also* Pain)
    altered reality and 129
    asthma 198
    double bind and 136
    fractional approach to 198
    resolution of 265
    substitution 227

Tactile
    cues 86
    dissociation and 147
    guidance 147
    trance awakening 147
Therapist (Hypnotherapist)
    attitudes 124
    life experiences 124
    patient response to 124
Therapy
    ripple effect of 261
    sudden 71, 72f
Thumbsucking
    double bind case of 262
Tic douloureux 220
Tichener, E. B. 21

Time distortion
  hypnosis and 37
  light trance and 149
Trance
  awakening 83, 88, 147, 184
  behavior 90, 135
  behavioral inevitabilities 184
  deep 110, 133
  deepening 90, 131, **248f**
  development 163
  double bind and 138
  everyday life 76
  focusing attention in 95
  hyper-alert 70
  indirect 250
  inducing 80, 101, 163
  learning 250
  light 110, 145, 149
  permissive 150
  phenomena 83
  ratifying 80, 84, 88, 253
  real vs. fake 86
  recognizing 87
  relaxed 84
  somnambulistic 231
  therapeutic 76
  time in 91
  unaffected 136, 174
  validity 149
  via memory
  without awareness 95, 149
Transference problem 49
Traumas 120
Truth 79

Ultradian cycles 85
Unconscious
  conscious and 162
  hypnosis 61f, **65**, 75
  reservoir of learning **65**
  utilization 75

Untutored boy 67
Utilization (Utilizing)
  appraoch **238f**
  authohypnosis 252f
  control and 272
  hypnosis 217
  ideas 75
  naturalistic 48
  patient behavior 104, **272**
  patient's framework **196f**
  patient's point of view 132
  perversity of human nature
    199
  religious beliefs 214
  resistance 167, 237, **238f**
  unconscious processes 75

Verbal
  explicit 150
  implicit 150
  mistakes 151
  nonverbal cues 240
Vocal
  inflection 242, 247
  intonation 242
  truth and 79
vonDedenroth, T. E. A. 28

Watzlawick, P. **54f**
Weakland, J. **40f**
Weitzenhoffer, A. 38, 52
Wundt, W. 21

Yes set
  facilitating 237, 240
Yogi 57

Zeig, J. **54f**

The book, <u>Healing in Hypnosis</u>, is accompanied
by a one-hour cassette tape recording, <u>Healing
in Hypnosis</u>:   <u>A Demonstration of Trance in
Everyday Life by Milton H. Erickson</u>.
Additional copies of the cassette are available
separately. Please send your check for $18.50
for a postpaid copy to Irvington Publishers, 551
Fifth Avenue, New York, NY 10176. Prepayment
is required. New York residents add sales tax.
Prices are subject to change without notice.